Making a Home

Assisted Living in the Community for Young Disabled People

JEN POWLEY

Roseway Publishing
an imprint of Fernwood Publishing
Halifax & Winnipeg

Development editing: Fazeela Jiwa
Copyediting and text design: Brenda Conroy
Cover design: Jess Koroscil, Housefires Design & Illustration
Photographs: Nicola Davison, Snickerdoodle Photography
Printed and bound in Canada

Published by Roseway Publishing
an imprint of Fernwood Publishing
2970 Oxford Street, Halifax, Nova Scotia, B3L 2W4
and 748 Broadway Avenue, Winnipeg, Manitoba, R3G 0X3
www.fernwoodpublishing.ca/roseway

Fernwood Publishing Company Limited gratefully acknowledges the financial support of the Government of Canada through the Canada Book Fund and the Canada Council for the Arts. We acknowledge the Province of Manitoba for support through the Manitoba Publishers Marketing Assistance Program and the Book Publishing Tax Credit. We acknowledge the Nova Scotia Department of Communities, Culture and Heritage for support through the Publishers Assistance Fund.

  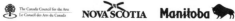

Library and Archives Canada Cataloguing in Publication
Title: Making a home: assisted living in the community for young disabled people / Jen Powley.
Names: Powley, Jen, author.
Identifiers: Canadiana (print) 20220498083 | Canadiana (ebook) 20220498091 | ISBN 9781773635958 (softcover) | ISBN 9781773636184 (EPUB) | ISBN 9781773636191 (PDF)
Subjects: LCSH: Group homes for people with disabilities—Canada. | LCSH: Young adults with disabilities—Housing—Canada. | LCSH: Youth with disabilities—Housing—Canada.
Classification: LCC HV1569.2.C3 P69 2023 | DDC 362.4/04850971—dc23

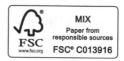

Making a Home

CONTENTS

For Barb and Bill, who believed in us,
Carrie and Kathleen, who worked tremendously hard to make this a reality,
Edward Edelstein, who believed in the vision,
Maria Medioli, who could imagine another way of doing things,
Vicky Levack, who demanded I try harder,
Tom Elliott, who I live for

ACRONYMS

ADLs   activities of daily living

ALS   amyotrophic lateral sclerosis

ARCs   adult residential centres

CCAs   continuing care assistants

CRPD   Convention on the Rights of Persons with Disabilities

DCS   Department of Community Services

DRC   Disability Rights Coalition of Nova Scotia

DSP   Disability Support Program

HRM   Halifax Regional Municipality

IL   independent living

ILNS   Independent Living Nova Scotia

MAID   medical assistance in dying

MS   multiple sclerosis

RRCs   regional rehabilitation centres

RRWs   residential resource workers

Chapter 1

THE PROBLEM

Visiting a Nursing Home

I was 37 when I first visited a nursing home with the thought, "Could I live here?" The place was Parkstone, owned and operated by Shannex. I knew it was a nursing home by its institutional smell. It must be the cleaning supplies they use because all institutions have the same reek of impersonality. Though it is meant to be a home, it does not smell like a home—either in a good way or a bad way. Maybe it was the hour at which I arrived, but it smelled neither like freshly baked cookies nor like mouldy damp towels. It smelled like nothing except cleaning chemicals.

My assistant should have known not to reverse that close to a wall. The headrest on my wheelchair has a metal pole sticking straight out behind it. Some people put tennis balls on pieces like that to contain the potential danger of the sharp edge, but I wanted my wheelchair to be adult-like. Maybe I should not have been so concerned about appearances, but I am not beyond that. So, when my assistant backed me up, I poked a hole right through the drywall. Thankfully, the nursing home did not sue for damages. I was sure they had a handyman on staff who could fix the drywall in an instant. Besides, it would look bad if they tried to sue me.

The rooms at Parkstone were not all bad. They were single rooms, which is a good start because they provide some privacy. I could make the room homey with the right quilt and curtains. But when I asked about their overnight guest policy, I was dismayed.

"My partner, Tom, stays overnight at least one night on the weekend. I was hoping you could guarantee him a cot." A cot wasn't as good as a regular bed; he wouldn't be able to put his large hand on my chest, cupping my two smaller hands. But at least I would be able to hear his soft snoring.

The person who was giving me the tour replied curtly, "I can appreciate that, but I am afraid the cots are first used for the relatives of people who are palliative."

At home, Tom kind of fits on my queen-size bed (he's a little too long for it), but in the nursing home I would have a twin bed. I can appreciate why cots go to the family members of people who are palliative, but why can't Parkstone purchase more cots? The government would be paying for my care, and I am sure Shannex's shareholders wouldn't even notice a few less dollars.

When I left the room, I looked sheepishly at the hole in the wall, then proceeded down the hall and out to my vehicle. Is there a "proper" reaction to having spent the afternoon visiting a nursing home? I had not read much on middle-aged women looking at nursing homes. I rolled out of the building, and I felt conflicted. Part of me wanted to scream and another part wanted to cry. I did neither, instead maintaining the cool demeanour of indifference. I have found that bottling up my emotions is the best way to be an appropriate role model for my numerous employees. I have had about ninety assistants over the years. I started needing an assistant when I went back to university to get my planning degree. I could drive neither my van nor my powerchair. I could not feed myself. It only got worse from there. That is the nature of progressive illnesses. When I hired university students to be my assistants, I had about ten on staff at any given time. I thought of myself as their wise older sister.

I thought if I talked to Tom about the issue he might have a solution. But I was worried that my emotions would affect the way he looks at me and about the bus ride he would eventually have to take to visit me. Instead, I let the emotions out as I cried myself to sleep. Other than this release, I kept it all inside. There, it only bothers me.

New to the Maritimes

I had been using some sort of homecare service since I moved to Nova Scotia for university from Alberta. When I got to Nova Scotia I looked up the different kinds of disability support programs. There are a host of homecare providers in Halifax, but the two most known are Northwood and Red Cross. I first hired Red Cross to watch me in the shower. They didn't actually watch me shower, but they ensured that I transferred successfully. They also ensured that my fingernails were kept at an acceptable length. I thought I should be ready if I needed more assistance. In Alberta I could get my mother to help. I had volunteered at a rowing club in Edmonton as a coxswain. I may not be able to row but I could sit forward and help steer and call to keep the rowers in unison. My mother was happy to drive me to rowing.

I had also taken accessible riding lessons in Alberta. When I decided to pursue accessible riding at the Bengal Lancers barn in downtown Halifax, Red Cross was already familiar with me. I thought they could walk me to the barn. However, when I called to confirm my spot at the Lancers, I was told quite insistently that a volunteer would come to the Dalhousie University residence where I was living to pick me up. It was only a few minutes away. I ended up in a relationship with that volunteer, and after my course finished I decided to stay in Nova Scotia to be with that person. When the relationship ended, I was alone for the nights. As a quadriplegic, being alone is not ideal.

I knew I didn't want to go into a nursing home, even though that might have seemed the most likely solution.[1] I hired a roommate who had to be on hand five nights out of seven. For the other two nights, I would either hire someone else or have a friend stay over. By this point I was having a Northwood homecare visit every morning to get me ready for my full-time job at the Ecology Action Centre. The costs of homecare should not have been more than a few hundred dollars a month, but mine were becoming astronomical. However, I kept myself out of a nursing home, my ultimate desire. If I'd had an accountant with more experience in disability tax matters, maybe we could have shaved a few dollars off the costs. I used my father as my accountant; he knew all the loopholes when it came to agriculture, but I might have been his only client with homecare.

I decided to go on the Department of Health and Wellness's Self-Managed Care Program.[2] You are expected to do all the advertising, hiring, training, firing, payroll, deductions, remittances and scheduling of your attendants. Because you are in charge of staffing, you determine the rate you pay the carers. As part of the program, you have to do a training course with the Department of Health and Wellness. People with disabilities should not need to have the skills to be their own bookkeepers, but in exchange you get a pot of funding, the amount of which depends on your needs. If you get the maximum amount and you pay minimum wage, you have enough for about six or seven hours of attendant care per day. That means the individual with a disability will be alone for 17 or 18 hours.

I was "lucky" that after an eight-year wait, I was approved to receive Flex funds from the Department of Community Services. With this funding I could afford to pay my workers more and for a greater number of hours. According to the Department's website,

> Flex provides individualized funding to participants living at home with their families or who live independently with support from their families or personal support networks.

That funding is used to:

a. purchase supports specific to a participant's disability-related needs and goals;

b. promote the participant's independence, self-reliance, and social inclusion; and

c. offer an alternative to, prevent or delay a participant's placement in a DSP-funded residential support option.[3]

I was primarily doing the latter.

I remember being on Access-A-Bus[4] and stopping in front of a retired fire station. At the stop, several wheelchair users were waiting for the bus. It was raining — not a heavy downpour but a smattering of large drops and persistent mist. I didn't know the exact mandate of the building, but I figured it must be some sort of group home.

I wonder how you get into this group home, I thought. I knew my condition was getting worse, not better. I knew living alone would one day no longer be an option. But I should have taken note that the other wheelchairs were all manual. I should have realized I wasn't in the same class as the others. Yes, we were all in wheelchairs, but we weren't in the same kind of wheelchairs.

A few days before, on September 23, 2006, I had sat outside for the Rolling Stones concert in the pouring rain, and my power wheelchair wouldn't turn on the next morning. Thankfully, I had just gotten it two days before, and it was still under the manufacturer's warranty. I was able to get it repaired, but I had to promise the sales rep that I would never, ever, take my chair out in the rain again.

I later checked out what was required for the group home on Oxford Street where I had seen the wheelchair users waiting in the rain. That group home only accepts levels 1 and 2, according to the grading scale developed by the Nova Scotia Department of Community Services. The details of the grades are somewhat obscure, but the higher the grade, the more disabled you are. While you might be able to transfer yourself from a wheelchair at a levels 1 and 2, by the time you get to level 4 you depend on a lift. Levels 1 and 2 are likely paraplegic. I was a level 4. So, I started to hunt for group homes that take level 4. There weren't any. Technically, group homes are supposed to take people with disabilities, but I couldn't find any that take people with disabilities as severe as my own.

Maybe we needed to start a new group home, I thought.

There were some examples I could draw from. Wheelchair user and quadriplegic Dan MacLellan had engineered the original Self-Managed Attendant Care Program with the help of Lois Miller, then director of the Metro Independent Living Resource Centre in Halifax. I had accessed this program for the pot of funding it provides. When it was taken over by the Department of Health and Wellness, it became known as the Self-Managed Care Program. With this program, Dan could get the assistance he needed and still live life how he wanted. He built a grand home in Halifax's North End, adjacent to the Hydrostone area. Dan only needed daily visits from a homecare worker. There was another unit with three bedrooms in the basement of his house which had a separate entrance. If he arranged it well, four people including himself could have 24-hour attendant coverage. I wanted to formalize the program and make 24-hour attendant care an option for people with severe physical disabilities in Nova Scotia.

I went to Dan MacLellan's house on Kane Street when it was for sale. It was winter and I remember the house as being well shovelled out. Unfortunately, Dan had passed away a few years earlier, and the relatives in charge of the house did not prioritize keeping any of the accessibility features. The elevator to access the floor with the master bedroom had not been maintained and inspected, and it was doubling as a closet. The washroom on the main floor had been renovated so that it was no longer accessible. Likewise, the counters in the kitchen had been raised, making them unsuitable for a wheel-chair user. In the basement, where there had been three units for wheelchair users, there were now five bedrooms. The changes were no doubt great for generating profit, but the house was no longer perfect for four people with severe physical disabilities.

I decided I did not want to enter a bidding war with other developers. It was a big lot. I may have made the wrong choice, but at the time it seemed the best decision for me. Rather than four people finding each other and pooling their funding to be able to live together, I wanted to formalize a program for people who needed more assistance but wanted to live in the community, so it could be an option for everyone. I wanted a concentrated effort to get young and middle-aged adults out of nursing homes.

In 2010, Canada signed the UN Convention on the Rights of People with Disabilities.[5] As a province of Canada, Nova Scotia falls under the terms of the Convention. When the UN's Special Rapporteur visited Nova Scotia in April 2019, she met with individuals with disabilities and their representative organizations, among others. In my presentation I talked about how the province wasn't giving individuals the choice of living situations guaranteed to them by the Convention.[6] I was later told by a lawyer that the UN Convention is aspirational and not enforceable under Canadian law. For something enforceable, you have to turn to human rights legislation. But Canada was trying to regain a seat on the UN Security Council, which it had lost in 2010. Living up to its commitments could not hurt its chances.[7]

On February 28, 2019, I presented a proposal to the Department of Community Services that detailed the cost of putting someone in a nursing home bed versus keeping them in their community. The numbers had been checked by Michelle Anderson, a researcher at Independent Living Nova Scotia (ILNS), and the cost of a nursing home placement was not substantially less than the cost of keeping the person in their community. I figured that if the option for living in the community was comparable to what government pays for nursing home beds, my proposal should be approved. The way I understood it, it must have just been easier for the Nova Scotia government to put people with severe physical disabilities in nursing homes — or continuing care homes as they are more politely called. In other jurisdictions, people with severe physical disabilities are not warehoused with people twice or three times their age. Instead, they are given the resources needed to live in the community and contribute to that community.

Unlike in Nova Scotia, in British Colombia, Alberta, Manitoba and Ontario, there are homes for people with severe physical disabilities where they can get the 24-hour care they require. I was lucky my parents could afford the $70,000 a year it costs to hire private attendants, but I knew they could not maintain this. My father was 76, yet still working full-time at his own private accounting practice. It is reasonable that he will one day retire. My mother, an elementary school counsellor and administrator, had retired, but she sold off a quarter section of our farmland on the Alberta prairies to finance my high-care needs.

My Situation

When I was diagnosed with multiple sclerosis at age 15, I did not think I would have a hard time finding a suitable living situation when I got older. I didn't know my multiple sclerosis would be progressive. I assumed my illness would be similar to that of my good friend's aunt. My friend's aunt had kids and a full-time job. She had to make sure she didn't get too tired, and she couldn't walk long distances, but other than that, she carried on a normal existence. It would not be that simple for me.

I was born in Alberta but moved to Nova Scotia after I completed my first university degree (I have four). There is a journalism after-degree program at the University of King's College in Halifax. I had been the editor of my university newspaper, and the program piqued my interest. I had wanted to go abroad for my university career, but I knew my diagnosis would make getting health insurance tricky.

Compared to Alberta, Nova Scotia is old. Halifax was founded in 1749, whereas Alberta was founded in 1905. So, going to Halifax was kind of like going to Europe — at least, that's what I told myself. I was already using a manual wheelchair when I moved to Nova Scotia, but we had not yet definitively established the kind of MS I had. There is no test for it; you simply have to wait and see. I had two different neurologists on different sides of the country, and maybe the doctors assumed my stressful life situation was causing my symptoms to worsen. Many people seem to think school is stressful. I thought it was a playground where I got to explore ideas. I could not have been happier.

I settled in Halifax. I found a boyfriend and began making my life. I fell in love with the city. I thought the pace more akin to my outlook and priorities. However, as my MS progressed, I was no longer able to work as a journalist. I couldn't go to an event and be sure that it would be accessible. I might have been able to ascertain that theatres were accessible, but they always place wheelchair users at the very front or very back of the auditorium. If there was a snowstorm, I knew the bus stop would be shovelled out eventually, but I didn't trust the allotted time given by the municipality. If there was a fire or flood, I likely couldn't be on hand providing commentary for a news story. I also was not able to take photographs. My waning eyesight made my choice of subject questionable. I thought I was taking photos of a woman toiling in the fields only to find out it was a scarecrow. Maybe I had picked the wrong profession.

I worked where I could. I ended up with a job at Metro Independent Living Resource Centre and later at the Nova Scotia

League for Equal Opportunities. Both jobs were disability related. My then boyfriend thought working for non-profits discredited my work. I knew work for people with disabilities is necessary. People with disabilities are at the bottom of the economic classes and often struggling. According to Statistics Canada's 2014 Longitudinal and International Study of Adults (LISA), "Persons with a disability accounted for approximately one-fifth of the overall population aged 25 to 64. Of these, 23% were in low income, compared with 9% of those without a disability."[8] Low-income rates vary by disability type. For example, the rate was 17% for those with a physical-sensory disability, 27% for those with a mental-cognitive disability, and 35% for those with a combination of both. If my boyfriend thought that disability made the work less valuable, then did he think the same about me? Was I only half a girlfriend because I couldn't walk?

Statistics Canada defines disability as a physical or mental impairment that is not accommodated by one's surrounding environment, making it more difficult to perform daily activities. This acknowledges that impairment does not have to result in disability if a person's physical and social environment fits their needs.

When my partner moved from his inaccessible apartment to one in a perfectly accessible new building, I didn't feel very disabled. He had to carry me up the stairs at his old apartment. It was great for a night or two of fooling around, but it wouldn't work in the long haul. Another problem arose if we were travelling cross country. I like pavement, but if I was on different ground, I again was thrown into the world of disability. My scrawny chicken arms couldn't push through grass.

Eventually, my relationship ended with the guy I had moved permanently to Nova Scotia to be with. This meant I had to adjust. I was lucky my family had the means to support me. I have learned that this may be the saving grace of being disabled. It is not something to do with me but the economic category I was born into. My mother was willing to purchase a condo with me. I could help with the down payment, and she had the credit history to get a mortgage. As my MS progressed, she took on more of the ownership role.

I found out that my MS was actually progressive, not because my doctor told me so but because I soon needed a powerchair. I didn't have the strength to push myself. It had nothing to do with the size of my biceps; my MS was just affecting me more.

I broke off another possible relationship when I met Tom. He was interesting. Now to get him interested in me. Tom had not seen my arms before we started to flirt, but that was not crucial to him. Because I was essentially a quadriplegic, I would joke that my arms were merely decorative. I wore shawls because I got cold and it was difficult to put on a sweater. Tom maintains his own apartment in Halifax's North End. He is willing to help me out whenever I need it. However, I knew I was not the only person with severe physical disabilities in the province who needed a home.

Sagewood

I stood at the front door with Tom waiting to be let into Sagewood. It was time for another meeting of the group of four disabled women now going under the name of Empowered. I usually referred to it as the group that met at Sagewood as our name seemed to change at the drop of a proverbial hat and I was horrible at keeping track of it. If we could get more political attention, maybe we would be more inclined to pick one name and stick with it.

Like at most nursing homes, you have to be approved by a staff member to be let in. It's a good security feature, but it's still annoying. My assistant, Emma, who had driven my van from Halifax, came up behind us as we waited to be buzzed in. The Empowered group had been initiated by Vicky Levack, Joanne Larade and

Melanie Gaunt, who had all found themselves in nursing homes after they could no longer be cared for at home without serious repercussions. Vicky was in her twenties and the others were in their forties, way too young to be placed in a home where most people were waiting for their demise.

I was a newcomer to their group. I was not yet in a nursing home but only because my family ensured I had the resources to live on my own. I was sure that I would be in a nursing home soon enough. I had already talked to my occupational therapist, a vivacious woman with blue hair, about which nursing home I should apply to go into. She said that Sagewood in Lower Sackville was the best. Unfortunately, it would mean a long bus ride for Tom, who doesn't drive.

Finally, a woman in dark red scrubs came to the door. "We are here for Joanne Larade's meeting," said Tom in his deep gravelly voice. "Come on in. She has the meeting room booked," said the cheerful attendant. Tom and I stopped to say hello to the yellow and green birds the nursing home keeps for the amusement of their residents. I would have to ask Joanne how it worked to have both a cat and birds at the residence. I suspected that the cat lived upstairs, and the birds lived downstairs, with any of the residents who have feline allergies. We made our way to the meeting room, where we had been before and knew the way. We were joined by Joanne, Vicky, Melanie and the notetaker Suzanne. Suzanne had brought coffee for the lot of us. I gave mine to Tom as I thought he needed it more than I did. I couldn't drink coffee anyhow, though I was not beyond putting it in my feeding tube.

We were trying to figure out how to convince politicians that nursing homes were not an appropriate home for people with severe physical disabilities. Little did we know that the municipal politician we had been talking to would one day end up as a cabinet minister in the provincial Conservative government.

Healthcare and social services are both provincial, so we lobbied provincial politicians, who were more accessible than federal ones. We had no real way of knowing if our talks with the politician would make a difference, but we hoped. The research is slim on younger people in nursing homes. Some good information is available from researchers Gloria M. Gutman[9] of Simon Fraser University and Michelle Hewitt,[10] co-chair of Disability Without Poverty in British Columbia. Jackie Egg, a researcher out of the Red Deer College in Alberta, turned to some research that was being done in Australia.[11] There is not much available nationally or even in the United States, though there is plenty on how to reform nursing homes for older adults.[12] What Gutman found, even back in her 1989 research, is that younger adults with chronic disabilities have differing needs than do seniors who are dying. Meagan Gilmore, in a recent article for *Broadview Magazine*, documented how some have called the warehousing of young people with disabilities in long-term care homes straight-up discrimination.[13]

A matter that's particularly important to me and others is sex. Younger adults with disabilities are often married or in common-law relationships, and many have young children. Conjugal visits are expected. For adults without permanent partners, sex is not off the table. Sex therapists may need to be part of the staffing complement. If we are truly treating the whole person, there should be money allotted for people to give sexual assistance to quadriplegics. A woman with quadriplegia may benefit from the use of a vibrator, but because she has no use of any of her appendages, she would need to hire someone to help her perform that task. The sexual health, especially of young people, should not be overlooked.

The manual for Sagewood only addresses sex in the negative, with a policy against abuse, but the Eden Philosophy, followed by Sagewood, might override this. The Eden Philosophy of care addresses the three plagues elders encounter, loneliness, helplessness and boredom, through principles of loving companionship and easy access to human and animal companionship. Though focused on seniors, the philosophy is appropriate for all people in care. In the spirit of the philosophy, sex should not only be tolerated but encouraged.

Younger adults in nursing homes primarily have multiple sclerosis, cerebral palsy and cervical spine injury (usually from motor vehicle accidents). The population of people under the age of 65 with severe physical disabilities is small but significant and increasing every year. According to Michelle Hewitt, "Statistics show that 7% of the residents of our long-term care homes are younger disabled adults in Canada, aged between 15 and 64."[14] In the US they make up about 14% of all nursing home admissions. Canada's rate may be lower because of population size.

As the healthcare system across all the provinces is encouraging older adults to stay at home longer with programs such as nursing assistance and cleaning services, the division between older adults with dementia and younger adults needing help with activities of daily living — both placed in nursing homes — is growing.

Other Provinces

If staying in Nova Scotia meant that I would be living in a nursing home, maybe Tom and I didn't want to live in Nova Scotia. That was our dilemma. I couldn't help but remember the 1982 song "Should I Stay or Should I Go?" by the Clash. There are plenty of other provinces to live in. Neither Tom nor I grew up on the East Coast, and thus our connection to the province is relatively shallow. Before moving to NS, Tom had lived in Winnipeg and spent time in the summer at his parents' cottage on East Blue Lake, Manitoba. (Tom's father was a school principal and his mother was a teacher's assistant.)

In Winnipeg, Ten Ten Sinclair is a housing development which came together in the 1970s as a place for younger Manitobans with physical disabilities. Luther Home Corporation, now known as Spinal Cord Injury Manitoba, a division of the Canadian Paraplegic Association, owns the complex. It provides suitable housing options and is flexible and ever changing. There are now four homes for people with severe physical disabilities. The homes are based on a Swedish concept called Fokus Housing:

> Fokus Housing represents the beliefs and views of individuals committed to a common goal and prepared to contribute to its maintenance on an ongoing basis. The goal incorporates the belief that every individual has a right to self-control, a free and independent lifestyle, self-management, and the exercising of rights and responsibilities inherent to every Canadian Citizen.[15]

But Tom's family is often not in Winnipeg. His parents spend their winters on Vancouver Island. Tom and I would depend on them for transportation to the lake. There is one accessible rental van in Manitoba. Manitoba was not on the top of the list, but it was not on the bottom either.

British Columbia was another option. Tom's parents have a timeshare on Vancouver Island and live there from January to March. It's seems to be the Winnipeg equivalent of going to Florida. Tom's friend Angela also lives on Vancouver Island. She works at a gallery and at a university. Tom and Angela still collaborate on art projects.

For over 25 years British Columbia has had the best, most established options for younger adults with physical disabilities.[16] The province has both group homes and nursing homes specifically for younger people with disabilities. And even in regular nursing homes in BC there are robust divisions for younger adults.

But it's still not clear what services they provide for quadriplegics who want sexual activity.

The problem with British Columbia is that the medical services I would need are found in Victoria whereas Tom's art partner lives elsewhere on the Island, as do his parents. Unlike in Nova Scotia, the population in the West is not considered to be elderly. According to Federal Retirees, "Seniors are the fastest-growing demographic in the country, and Nova Scotia is 4 per cent above the national average. With over 21 percent of its population aged 65 or older, the province has the third-highest proportion of seniors in Canada."

I was initially scared of the idea of living on an island given climate change and the rise in sea levels, but in Halifax we are right on the ocean and I should probably be more concerned about climate change right here. Nova Scotia is essentially an island connected by a sliver of low-lying land to New Brunswick. There is a mountain on Vancouver Island. Nova Scotia has a ski hill that is just that, a hill. I reconsidered staying in Halifax.

BC may be further ahead than the East Coast because of the weather. It is amenable to being outdoors in the winter. In February of 2022 the average temperature was 4.4 degrees Celsius in Vancouver. In Halifax it was -4 degrees, and for purposes of comparison, it was -19.6 degrees in Winnipeg.

I was born in Alberta. My father lives in Vegreville. My sisters live in Leduc and Calgary. My mother resides in Vegreville but after her mother passed away last summer, she and her partner have been looking to relocate. They were looking at BC but the floods and the fires because of climate change have made them reconsider.

My mother stayed in Vegreville because she was there primarily to look after my grandmother. On his deathbed my grandfather had asked my mother to look after my grandmother. He knew he was dying and would not be there for her. My grandmother adopted the same outlook as my grandfather, her husband, had. I would talk about going to other countries. He would look at me in his unflinching manner and ask me with all solemnity, "Why? What are you looking for that you don't have right here?" As a teenager, I was at a loss for words. I didn't know how to justify my desire to see other lands and other ways of interacting.

The government of Alberta does provide support for people with a wide range of issues, issues that could qualify them for placement in a nursing home. They provide round-the-clock assistance to those who have the ability to direct their own care.[17] I have not applied because I am currently a resident of Nova Scotia, and it is difficult to know if you would qualify for any particular program unless you know the intake coordinator and their superiors.

In Calgary, there is Horizon Housing Association[18] and the Accessible Housing Organization.[19] Though they have over 1000 accessible units for people of low income, I could not apply with a Nova Scotia address and documentation. I would first need to move to Alberta and reside there for three months before I would be eligible as a resident.

Although it is great that the country of Canada provides for its citizens, the division of power between the federal and provincial governments means there are 13 different systems to work through if you include the territories.

Developers

Since it was improbable that the politicians would listen to our lobbying, and it seemed not ideal to move to another province, I began thinking about just starting our own group home in Nova Scotia. How hard could it be?

I needed a developer. The only one I really knew had been on the province's Built Environment Standards Development

Committee. I had tried to talk with him, but he told me he was really busy and didn't have time for my little concerns. Then I remembered that I did know one other, the developer of the apartment building I used to live in. I called his office, but they were not particularly helpful. I know of other developers, but not well enough to ask a favour of them. So, I did what I do with every other problem I have. I talked to Tom.

Tom told me that the building his office was in was owned by the biggest developer in Halifax's North End, Edward Edelstein. His company was called Eco-Green, and their mission was to "Build and renovate homes and workplaces that are low energy, durable, and low maintenance." That was exactly what I needed.

Tom arranged a meeting between me and Mr. Edelstein. I knew my voice was not strong enough to lead the meeting. Tom said he would be there, and I asked him to speak for me. He was willing to do whatever was needed. I thought I should get treats for the first meeting with Mr. Edelstein. If I learned anything from my time working in an office, it is that meetings always go better when treats are involved. Maybe that is not earth-shattering news, but it is true. I stopped at the LF Bakery and bought chocolate croissants and a few coffees. I picked up cream and sugar. I knew Tom only took cream in his coffee, but there were going to be other people at the meeting.

Edward Edelstein was receptive to the idea of an apartment with four bedrooms for people with severe physical disabilities. He couldn't believe that something like this did not already exist. He agreed to put the unit on the main floor of the building he was already constructing near Tom's office. He got his own staff to draw up a schematic for the living space. He wanted to reserve the front portion of the main floor for a business storefront. The floor under our prospective unit was going to be a daycare. This was great because we could share services like smoke detectors.

When I met with the Department of Community Services about the proposal I was presenting for the Shared Attendant Project, I wanted to have my proverbial ducks in a row. I was trusting that the four-person scheme worked out for the Self-Managed Care Program, which had been studied by the Metro Independent Living Resource Centre, was cost effective and that it still held weight with the provincial government. I thought, they could give us funding for the build, and we could continue to have the support of Self-Managed Care.

I brought Carrie Ernst, the executive director of Independent Living Nova Scotia, on board. I thought that, with Edward, we made a good team. We presented to the Department, and they were impressed. I had joked with the director of Disability Services prior to the meeting. I used the fact that I am legally blind to my advantage. I do not get nervous; I cannot tell who people are. It is a bit of a safety cushion. Our initial proposal is reproduced below.

Shared Attendant Project

Our Proposal

We are asking the Province of Nova Scotia to invest in a *small options home for four persons with severe physical disabilities* at a rate equivalent or greater to what is currently being provided for small options homes for people with intellectual disabilities.

Residents of the home would have 24-hour shared attendant care. Funding for the small options home provided must be based on an independent evaluation of each resident's physical and independence needs. The home must include Jen Powley as a resident. The other three people with severe physical disabilities can be decided upon jointly by Independent Living Nova Scotia and the Department of Community Services.

The small options home will *cost roughly $1.4 million over three years*. This is dependent on specific needs of the clients. The builder requires $12,000 for design to accommodate those needs.

Current situation

It is important to note that in the current environment, the health system is supporting many individuals with high care needs in hospitals. The cost of a hospital bed is over $1,300 per day which, for four people over three years, would equate to $5.7 million.

A nursing home bed costs $250 per day which, for four people over three years equates to $1.1 million, the quality of life and contribution to society are greatly reduced in that option.

Of course, in the case of a nursing home bed you must also factor in wait times which are greater than six months. Many seniors waiting for a bed are being cared for in hospitals at great expense. By moving younger, physically disabled people from nursing homes into more appropriate care facilities — like small options homes — beds are freed up in the nursing home, and on in-patient wards in our adult hospitals.

At present, there are currently 240 Nova Scotians between the ages of 18 and 60 living in nursing homes. A person with a high-level of physical care needs in Nova Scotia will be put in a nursing home, whether they are young or old. Alternatively, they are offered a maximum of $3,900 per month for Self-Managed Care. That amount would only provide 6.6 hours of care per day at $19.18 per hour. $3,900 per month equates to $125.80 per day in a month with 31 days. This total does not include CRA deductions made as an employer. In the case where a person has severe mobility and voice limitations, it also requires that the support amount includes the cost of hiring someone to complete employee scheduling and payroll. *If an individual agrees to self-manage*, all publicly funded home care is discontinued.

Details of the home

The small options home would operate as a pilot project with yearly financial reports and assessments being done by the staff and residents, as well as by the Department of Community Services. The format for these reports will be worked out in a separate document. A small options home for people with physical disabilities would require that residents have an opportunity to provide substantial input into the day-to-day operations of the home, including devising a code of conduct. *The home is proposed to be located on 2165 Gottingen Street, in a multi-storey, energy efficient building.* Eco Green Homes is in the midst of construction and has agreed to incorporate the small options home into the building, should funding be made available. This location is within an area that makes access to community events by wheelchair, car, bus, or walking, convenient.

The small options home will be given a three-year trial with an option to renew indefinitely.

How does this support existing provincial goals

The *Nova Scotia Accessibility Act* aims to make Nova Scotia fully accessible by 2030. This assumes that people with disabilities can be active members of society. For certain individuals with physical disabilities, being an active member of society is not possible without almost full-time attendant care. *This proposal would offer a solution aligned with the positive goals within the legislation that could evolve from a pilot to a solution for many other Nova Scotians.*

Models from other cities

To be active members of society, people with disabilities need homes that are affordable and part of the community. Here are a couple of projects in other provinces:

1. Fokus Housing and Services in Winnipeg is based upon a Swedish concept that facilitates individuals living with physical disabilities to live in the community by providing wheelchair accessible suites with attendant care services, housekeeping, and meal preparation.

2. Inclusion in Calgary was designed for adults over the age of 18 who require some assistance with their daily lives, but also value autonomy and independence.

Who we are

Independent Living Nova Scotia (ILNS) is a charitable organization operating in Halifax. It is one of 24 independent living organizations affiliated with Independent Living Canada. The current Executive Director is Carrie Ernst and the Special Projects Coordinator is Michelle Anderson. ILNS has been fortunate enough to get funding from the Department of Community Services to develop a business model for shared attendant care. They see the pilot as a way of ensuring the process moves ahead.

Jennifer Powley is a 41-year-old woman who is quadriplegic due to progressive multiple sclerosis. She is a former director of the Nova Scotia League for Equal Opportunities, and a former staff member of Independent Living Resource Centre. She holds a degree in Urban Planning and was recently awarded the 2018 Margaret and John Savage First Time Author Nonfiction Book Award for her memoir *Just Jen*. Jen has paired with ILNS and Eco Green Homes on this project.

EcoGreen Homes, incorporated in 2001, is a Halifax based design-build construction company employing a licensed architect, designers, carpenters, a certified welder, and a cabinet maker. They have agreed to take on the design and construction of the small options home and will house it in one of their ongoing builds. Their design office is located at 2159 Gottingen Street and their 7000 sq. ft shop is at the rear of 2019 Gottingen. Recently completed design-build projects include: Compass Distilleries, 2533 Agricola, LF Bakery, 2063 Gottingen, the Lower Gym at Seven Bays Bouldering, 2019 Gottingen, Music Nova Scotia, Tiny Lab Daycare, Leave Out Violence, The Centre for Art Tapes, and 6 apartments at 2169/71 Gottingen, Ratinaud and the Kitchen Table, EGH's Office and 3 apartments at 2157/9 Gottingen Street, The Benches on Barrington and Duke St, Shakespeare by The Sea Theatre, 5480 Point Pleasant Park Drive and their stage/berm in the Cambridge Battery, and two student duplexes on LeMarchant Street.

No More Warehousing Event

I wanted to hit the Department of Community Services with a one-two punch. One was the presentation of the proposal and two was an event held at the library the same evening. The event, put on by the organization No More Warehousing, which I co-founded with a friend and former employee, Emma Cameron, would feature the lived experience of three younger people who were residing in nursing homes. Edward chatted with me in the lobby of Nelson Place, where the Community Services offices are, about our event. He planned on attending that evening.

Several people we had presented our proposal to attended the event. At least I had raised their interest. I don't know if a lot of other people who came were curious about young people living in continuing care facilities, or if they were as incensed as I was about the province's management techniques.

"We aren't allowed any more people. A library representative just came by and told me the room is at the maximum for fire regulations," Tom told me calmly.

I was elated. An event about young people in nursing homes drew a packed house. The director of Disability Supports and a colleague of hers from the Department of Community Services were sitting in the front row. I couldn't have made a stronger statement.

"We should put a sign on the door explaining the situation and telling them that there will be a video of the event on YouTube under the heading No More Warehousing Panel in a couple of days," I replied to Tom, seeming to take it all in stride. I was wondering where we would get paper in this digital age. I knew where my smartphone was, but finding a pen and paper was trickier. The encee for the evening (my occupational therapist, Cher Smith) leaned in and said, "That's great news, Jen."

Finally, Cher asked the room to settle down because we would begin in a minute. After an intro from me about the province's and the country's commitments, I posed the troubling question:

The directory of nursing homes and residential care facilities put out by the Department of Health and Wellness states that "Nursing Homes are an option for people who have difficulty performing everyday tasks, such as dressing or bathing, and are appropriate for those who are medically stable yet have nursing needs beyond home care." If nursing homes are an option, what other options are available for people with severe physical disabilities? There is Self-Managed Care, administered by the Department of Health and Wellness. If you qualify for that program, the department will provide funding that will cover 6 or 7 hours of attendant care per day. What is an individual like me supposed to do for the remaining 17 or 18 hours? For me, it looks like a nursing home might be the only option. According to the 2016 census, there are 240 Nova Scotians between the ages of 18 and 60 living in nursing homes. In reality, this number is likely higher, because not everyone living in a nursing home fills out the census.

After that, we were on to the main show. There was a video from Catherine Frazee, a professor emerita in the School of Disability Studies at Ryerson University, who is living in Baxter's Harbour, near Kentville, NS, on the Bay of Fundy. She sees nursing homes as part of the disability Gulag. Nova Scotians with disabilities are not asking for a better Gulag. They want the right to choose where they live and are demanding to have the services they need and deserve.

Next was Claire McNeil, a lawyer with the Disability Rights Coalition of Nova Scotia, which had just taken the province to court over the Emerald Hall case.[20] That case concerned three people with intellectual disabilities who were institutionalized rather than given homes in the community. McNeil explained the difference between the aspirational goals of the UN, which the government committed to, versus the human rights legislation, which, in contrast, is legally enforceable through the courts. After her eloquent speech, there was a commentary from Carrie Ernst, the executive director of Independent Living Nova Scotia. This was followed by a video from Bonnie Sheer Klein, the director of *Shameless: The Art of Disability* (2006), available on Amazon Prime Video. Sheer Klein complimented us on our imaginative proposal.

She reminded us to think of the whole person, not just the physical care but the emotional and spiritual well-being, and she reminded us that people with disabilities know what they need. Following Sheer Klein was the parent of a young woman who had no choice but to place her daughter, Ellen, in a nursing home after her own health failed and she could no longer perform the activities of daily living for her daughter.

Lastly, three younger adults, Joanne Larade, Vicky Levack and Melanie Gaunt, described their lives in nursing homes. Joanne spoke about what living in a long-term care facility with people twice her age, many of whom had dementia, taught her about herself. She learned she was exceedingly patient and incredibly strong. The residents became her new family, and she mourned the loss of each one. Vicky Levack, sexuality and disability advocate, was forced to enter a nursing home to ensure she would receive the 24-hour care she required because her step-mother was feeling trapped as the care workers didn't show up reliably. At a nursing home, Vicky could be assured that her basic needs would be met. She said it was important to separate people with physical disabilities from those whose cognitive ability was impaired. Melanie Gaunt, master of arts in organizational communication and a researcher at Dalhousie University, spoke about the drawbacks of living in long-term care. She said that young adults are anywhere between the ages of 18 and 64. She was on a special diet, which the long-term care facility had a problem dealing with and required her to request different meals. She also had to put in a request to get bathed more than once a week. Her requests were not extraordinary, but in a system where there are only 13 workers for a floor of clients, her requests looked beyond possible.

Questions followed. Edward Edelstein, the developer, asked if the community could help fund the development of the unit. I imagine that he was looking for any way possible to make the unit a reality. He had the space in one of his buildings; now he just needed the capital. He was fully on board for developing a home in the community for younger adults with severe physical disabilities, but he was not used to the snail's pace at which the provincial government operates.

What Edelstein may not have realized is that the provincial government has put young people with severe physical disabilities in institutions for longer than any one person can remember. There are currently 1900 people waiting for small options homes, and that is only people with intellectual disabilities. There are approximately 300 people with severe physical disabilities between 18 and 64 who have been inappropriately placed in nursing homes. Add to that the people in regional residential care facilities and the number only grows.[21]

The Dignity of Risk

No one remembers when Nova Scotia didn't put individuals with severe physical disabilities in nursing homes. The current director of the Disability Support Program at the Department of Community Services, Maria Medioli, wrote in an email to me on March 16, 2022, that no one in her office knew a time when people at a level 4 support need didn't get put in nursing homes. Medioli is new blood; she has a varied background, including everything from accounting to planning to social work. Maybe it is her fresh outlook that let her consider our proposal with an open mind. She was not stuck on stale ideas. She hadn't been indoctrinated into the view that people with disabilities were sick.

The book *The Principle of Normalization in Human Services,* by Wolf Wolfensberger, states that "a highly visible portion of human management concerns itself with individuals whom the public, or a significant segment of it, views as 'deviant.'"[22] Wolfensberger hits the nail on the head: people with a disability are considered deviant in that they deviate from the norm. "Atypical" could be another word to describe this. Wolfensberger writes, "It clearly must be kept in mind that deviancy is of our own making; it is in the eyes of the beholder." While someone who is not disabled might view the activities of daily living that are required by a person with a disability as demeaning, the person who is disabled knows that they are required to maintain their healthy existence. For example, I have routine bowel care appointments where a nurse sticks a finger up my rectum. It is not fun, but it is a way to remove the feces. It would be nicer if I could void normally, but I can't.

It makes sense that, if the Department of Health and Wellness is involved, they would put people with severe physical disabilities — no matter what their age — in facilities the department was familiar with, like long-term care facilities. Simple. The Department of Health and Wellness knows that long-term care facilities have the personnel to look after the complex needs of these individuals, who are seen as having a health condition. Their needs are beyond the scope of the Department of Community Services, which does have disability support programs, but only for disabilities that do not require 24-hour care. The government can provide 24-hour residential facilities, but does not have the ability to provide 24-hour care. It is a slight distinction, but one that has huge implications.

An important part of disability rights discourse is self-determination: the argument goes that, despite needing assistance and care, the person should be able to make their own decisions. This notion is often referred to as the "dignity of risk." It simply means that part of self-determination is the right to take reasonable risks, which is crucial to maintaining dignity. As we know, there are always risks in any situation. The dignity of risk is a matter of being able to choose the risks you will take. The dignity of risk is important for caregivers, elderly people, children and people with disabilities. And it's part of living in community rather than being institutionalized.

My partner Tom and I have been together for thirteen years. However, we made the decision not to get married because that creates legal obligations that we did not want to be bound by. We do not live together in a common-law relationship; Tom maintains his own apartment. Unfortunately, the havoc wreaked by COVID-19 put a kink in our best-laid plans. The nurse I got through a homecare agency was working in the hospital and therefore was possibly exposed to COVID-19. I couldn't risk being exposed. My nurse's girlfriend also worked in the COVID-19 unit. As a result, my partner took over morning homecare duties. Many people have children or parents or a partner who will look after them, but many people do not have people in their lives who can take over their care, and the system should not depend on them.

Notes

1. Joseph Shapiro, "A New Nursing Home Population: The Young," *NPR*, December 10, 2010. npr.org/2010/12/09/131912529/a-new-nursing-home-population-the-young.
2. Government of Nova Scotia, "Self-Managed Care," n.d. novascotia.ca/dhw/ccs/self-managed-care.asp.
3. Department of Community Services, "Flex Program," Government of Nova Scotia, n.d. https://novascotia.ca/coms/disabilities/FlexProgram.html.
4. Halifax Regional Municipality, "Access-A-Bus," November 29, 2021. halifax.ca/transportation/halifax-transit/access-a-bus.
5. Government of Canada, "Promoting Rights of Persons with Disabilities," January 30, 2020. https://www.international.gc.ca/world-monde/issues_development-enjeux_developpement/human_rights-droits_homme/rights_disabilities-droits_handicapees.aspx?lang=eng; United Nations, "Convention on the Rights of Persons with Disabilities (CRPD)" n.d. un.org/development/desa/disabilities/convention-on-the-rights-of-persons-with-disabilities.html#Fulltext.
6. Jennifer Henderson, "Report: Nova Scotia Failing to Meet Its Commitment to De-Institutionalize People with Disabilities," *Halifax Examiner*, July 20, 2021. https://www.halifaxexaminer.ca/government/province-house/

report-nova-scotia-failing-to-meet-its-commitment-to-de-institutionalize-people-with-disabilities/.
7. Ola Mohajer, "Six Steps Canada Must Take to Win a UN Security Council Seat," *Open Canada*, May 13, 2019. opencanada.org/six-steps-canada-must-take-win-un-security-council-seat.
8. Statistics Canada, "Longitudinal and International Study of Adults." 2014. https://www.statcan.gc.ca/en/survey/household/5144.
9. Gloria M. Gutman, *Younger Adults in Long-Term Care Facilities: A Review of the Literature Concerning Their Characteristics and Environmental Design, Staffing and Programming Needs*, Literature review, Gerontology Research Centre at Simon Fraser University, 1989. researchgate.net/profile/Gloria-Gutman/publication/277799870_Younger_adults_in_long-term_care_facilities_a_review_of_the_literature_concerning_their_characteristics_and_environmental_design_staffing_and_programming_needs/links/56a6509d08ae2c689d39e600/Younger-adults-in-long-term-care-facilities-a-review-of-the-literature-concerning-their-characteristics-and-environmental-design-staffing-and-programming-needs.pdf.
10. Michelle Hewitt, "How Does a Foucauldian Genealogical Approach Enhance the Study of Long-Term Care through a Critical Disability Lens?" *Societies,* 12, 3: 73 (2022). https://doi.org/10.3390/soc12030073.
11. Jackie Egg, "What Factors Contribute to Quality of Life for Young Disabled Adults Who Live in Long Term Care?" BCR (Brief constructed response), Red Deer College, 2008.
12. Gloria M. Gutman, Keith G. Anderson and Judith B. Killam, *Younger Adults with Severe Physical Disabilities in the Capital Region*, Literature review, Gerontology Research Centre at Simon Fraser University, 1995. https://summit.sfu.ca/_flysystem/fedora/sfu_migrate/555/GRC_020.pdf.
13. Meagan Gillmore, "Some Young Adults with Disabilities Are Stuck in Long-Term Care. They Say That's Discrimination," *Broadview Magazine*, November 15, 2021. broadview.org/young-people-with-disabilities-long-term-care.
14. Michelle Hewitt, "How Does a Foucauldian Genealogical Approach."
15. Ten Ten, "What Is Fokus Housing and Services?" n.d. tenten.mb.ca/housing/fokus/.
16. Government of British Columbia, Canada, "Care Options and Costs," n.d. gov.bc.ca/gov/content/health/accessing-health-care/home-community-care/care-options-and-cost.
17. Alberta Health Services, "Programs & Services: Designated Supportive Living Level 4," n.d. albertahealthservices.ca/findhealth/service.aspx?Id=1067277&facilityId=1057554; Government of Alberta, Canada, "Community Access for People in Continuing Care," n.d. alberta.ca/community-access-continuing-care.aspx.
18. Horizon Housing, "Referring Partners," n.d. https://www.horizonhousing.ab.ca/our-partners/service-providers/.

19. Accessible Housing, "Vision, Mission & Values," n.d. https://accessible-housing.ca/vision-mission-values/.
20. Disability Rights Coalition of Nova Scotia, "DRC Complaint of Systemic Discrimination before the Nova Scotia Court of Appeal (2019–2021)," n.d. disabilityrightscoalitionns.ca/drc-complaint-of-systemic-discrimination-before-the-nova-scotia-court-of-appeal.
21. Disability Rights Coalition of Nova Scotia, "Road to Inclusion by 2023: Come with Us," January 16, 2022. https://www.disabilityrightscoalitionns.ca/road-to-inclusion-by-2023-come-with-us/. Some of the information in this paragraph also comes from a personal email from Maria Medioli on March 16, 2022.
22. Wolf Wolfensberger, Nirje Bengt, Simon Olshansky et al., *The Principle of Normalization in Human Services*, Toronto: National Institute on Mental Retardation, 1986.

Chapter 2

LIVING WITH A DISABILITY

The Shared Attendant Pilot Program

For our proposed Shared Attendant Program to go ahead, both the Department of Community Services and the Department of Health and Wellness needed to be involved. Neither department saw providing the program as entirely their responsibility. This was because the proposal deals with ensuring that people with severe physical disabilities who require 24-hour support, who are often housed in nursing homes (funded by Health and Wellness), are given the opportunity of living in their community (funded by Community Services). Government deems the needs of people requiring 24/7 care to be complex, but the only thing complicated about their needs is the way these needs are going to be funded.

Society considers people with complex care needs as "sick," but an infant has the same care needs, and they are not thought to be ill. There are no expectations that babies can do activities of daily living (ADLs) themselves, but everything is viewed differently when it is an adult who cannot perform those activities on their own.

"I need help with all of my ADLs and I'm very reliant on physical care. I can't do many physical things for myself," says Vicky Levack, an adult who has been labelled as having complex care needs. Therefore, Vicky has been living in a long-term care facility, otherwise known as a nursing home. The Shared Attendant Program we proposed to the Department of Community Services offers the services that Vicky needs while letting her remain in the community.

The problem is that a service like community homecare is typically one-on-one and is normally provided by a certified care attendant, like in the case of nursing homes or with Northwood and Red Cross, and the cost is expensive. There is a shortage of certified care attendants, and their level of compensation matches their level of training. The Shared Attendant Program, on the other hand, does not demand the use of certified care attendants or use a one-on-one system like traditional homecare. It's a pilot program because the government is trying it out; the benefits are technically still unproven.

No specialized training is needed for the care of Vicky or myself as we have similar deficits. If I hadn't had the ingenuity to figure out another way of doing things, and if I didn't have the partner I do and access to money sometimes, I would also have been placed in a nursing home. All that is needed for our "elaborate" care is common sense, basic knowledge of anatomy, compassion, and the utmost care and observation. I happen to be training a new assistant as I write this, and when I asked him how it was going, he replied, "It is not rocket science." I have been able to survive quite well using university students as attendants. I have gotten a homecare service or my partner to do morning care, which involves the washing up and cleaning if I have any accidents overnight. Like Vicky, I cannot perform any of my own activities of daily living, but I am not sick, and my needs are not particularly complicated — unless being cleaned and fed are complex.

Independent Living Nova Scotia (ILNS) is in favour of providing options within the community for people with "complex" needs. They brought together two people who desperately wanted to change how long-term care in Nova Scotia works with the executive director of Disability Supports, Joe Rudderham. I was one of those people and the other was Kevin Penny, a quadriplegic from an automobile accident while he was still in high school. He had a partner, so he was okay for the moment, but I am sure he had the same fears that I had. What happens if my partner gets sick or there is a family emergency? Both of these things have happened with Tom in the past couple of years.

Before ILNS and I could go forward with the Shared Attendant Program, some basic research into the costs and potential benefits needed to be completed. I had proposed that four individuals with severe physical disabilities could share a resource worker. This type of worker is used by other residential homes, such as group homes for people with autism or intellectual disabilities. We thought we could rent two apartments on the same floor. We didn't want to deal with elevator hassles. The two units would be linked with a baby monitor. I was unaware of this type of worker until we began to advertise. I thought we would be looking for a certified care attendant. Carrie and ILNS were in charge of the program details; I was the big picture thinker. A basic first-aid course and a reminder to call 911 if there is ever a health emergency are all that we required. The Shared Attendant Program would always have at least one worker on-site, more during the morning rush. Participants would get about 10 hours a month of support in their community, for example, for getting groceries. I had learned about meal planning when I was still in my mother's home, but we couldn't assume that program participants would have that knowledge — they might be coming from an institution where all that was done for them.

The Shared Attendant Program needed a business model. Rudderham had a pot of funding for special projects up to $20,000. This would be enough for ILNS to hire someone to do research on programs that already exist in Canada and how a similar program might work in Nova Scotia. ILNS applied for and was awarded the

JEN POWLEY

funding, with the deadline for the project completion being June 2019. That timing may have been part of the reason why the decision on my proposal was so late.

The next time I met with Disability Supports, Rudderham's job as executive director had been filled by Maria Medioli, and according to Carrie Ernst from ILNS, "Maria really got it."

Whether the individual was disabled through an accident like Kevin, a medical illness like me, or a congenital condition like Harriet McBryde Johnson or Vicky Levack, we all enjoy the same pleasures as any other person. We all want to live in our own homes with our own rules. As Johnson states in *Too Late to Die Young,* "We enjoy pleasure other people enjoy, and pleasures peculiarly our own. We have something the world needs."[1]

At the same time, we are acutely aware, as Johnson says, that "all placement is determined not by our needs, nor by our desires, but by what the government will pay for. Public policies rob us of freedom and security just as surely as would a late-night knock on the door by the secret police."[2] Johnson was writing about the United States, but the situation is similar in Canada. People with disabilities (unless they are independently wealthy) are expected to survive in a broken system.

The Medicalization of Disability

My partner Tom is a type 1 diabetic. I tried to encourage him to check off that he has a disability when he was applying for a job with the municipality but was met a lot of resistance. It wasn't until I "proved" that diabetes was legitimately a disability according to federal tax guidelines[3] that he relented. The way in which disability is defined may be at the root of the problem of how society sees people with disabilities.[4] The US Centers for Disease Control and Prevention defines disability as "any condition of the body or mind (impairment) that makes it more difficult for the person with the condition to do certain activities (activity limitation) and interact with the world around them (participation restrictions)."[5] There are many types of disabilities, such as those that affect a person's vision, movement, thinking, remembering, learning, communicating, hearing, mental health and social relationships.

I was on the Built Environment Standards Development Committee, one of the first committees Nova Scotia struck in the effort to become accessible by 2030. (I qualified to be on the committee because I am a licensed urban planner.) The committee worked to develop accessibility criteria for both public and private buildings (though the regulations would not affect private homes). We developed the recommendations for seven types of disability, but sometimes the needs of the groups were contradictory. The Deaf and the Hard of Hearing prefer bright lighting, but people who are autistic prefer muted lighting. This left us in a quandary. We recommended that the lighting have two different settings, bright and muted.

Most North Americans have bought into the concept of medicalization (at least they had until COVID-19 in 2019 when trust in health authorities started to wane and medical misinformation spread far and wide). Medicalization is the belief that anything can be solved with the application of the medical model. Zoe Swaine, writing in the *Encyclopedia of Clinical Neuropsychology*, explains that the medical model is "a model of health which suggests that disease is detected and identified through a systematic process of observation, description, and differentiation, in accordance with standard accepted procedures, such as medical examinations, tests, or a set of symptom descriptions."[6] Swaine presents three major criticisms of the model:

(1) it supports the false notion of dualism in health, whereby biological and psychological problems are treated separately;

(2) it focuses too heavily on disability and impairment rather than on individual's abilities and strengths; and

(3) it encourages paternalism within medicine rather than patient empowerment.

Science may hold the position of highest authority, but it must be tempered by humanity. "Medical treatment should be the servant of genuine human caring, never its master," says the Eden Alternative, which is a philosophy of person-driven care geared primarily toward elders but also applicable to young people with disabilities.[7]

People with disabilities are seen as broken because they do not conform to the ideals of the medical model. According to Simi Linton in *The Disability Studies Reader*, "the medicalization of disability casts human variation as deviance from the norm, as pathological condition, as deficit, and, significantly, as an individual burden and personal tragedy." *The Disability Studies Reader* points to how disability is put on the individual rather than on the social construct which makes impairment an issue. It is the system we live in that is broken. The author of the chapter goes on to say:

> As typically used, the term disability is a linchpin in a complex web of social ideals, institutional structures, and government policies. As a result, many people have a vested interest in keeping a tenacious hold on the current meaning because it is consistent with the practice and policies that are central to their livelihood or their ideologies.[8]

We have constructed our current system with this sort of medicalization. It would be unprecedented to look at it differently. The medicalization of disability got society into a certain mindset, which is hard to break. Thus, changing the system is slow and almost impossible, but it can be done. It takes courage and a lot of patience.

Further in the chapter, Linton writes, "The degree and significance of an individual's impairment is often less of an issue than the degree to which someone identifies as disabled."[9]

Being medicalized may impact the way you perceive yourself, and thinking of yourself as different from the rest of humanity can impact your sense of self-worth. If you see yourself as unlovable due to your differences, then you have already cut yourself off from interacting with others. Roy Baumeister, in *The Paradox of Disability*, writes, "Exclusion may be partly or wholly self-imposed, insofar as people with disabilities may themselves avoid some kinds of social interactions for several reasons: because they dislike being the object of others' pity, or they fear rejection or other negative reactions, or because the persons with disabilities feel embarrassed or ashamed about their own incapacities."[10] Maybe because I was not born with my disability, but acquired it later in life, I am not likely to look down on myself. But I felt very differently when I was younger. I never thought I would ever find a partner, for example. I think it depends on the day you ask.

The Indigenous Peoples of Turtle Island do not have a medical model, as far as I can tell from research and conversation. Nicole Inesse-Nash, in an article entitled "Disability as a Colonial Construct: The Missing Discourse of Culture in Conceptualizations of Disabled Indigenous Children," says there is no word for disability in many of the Indigenous languages. She writes that in Anishinaabe culture people are named for the gifts they bring to the community. There is no need for the word disability because the focus is on what you can do rather than on what you can't do.[11] This is an exciting way to view the individual, not by their deficiencies but by their strengths. Ineese-Nash writes, "The label of disability is a colonial construct that conflicts with Indigenous perspectives of community membership and perpetuates assimilation practices which maintain colonial harm." If colonially governed

North America had done that, maybe we wouldn't have built such inaccessible cities. But because we did, we now need the initiative to try to correct our wrongs.

Dustin Galer, in *Work Disability in Canada: Portraits of a System,* writes, "Indigenous cultures primarily defined disability as an imbalance between mind, body and spirit that affected participation and relationships within the community." He continues; "Mental and physical disabilities were sometimes seen as a divine gift or accepted as a natural part of aging. Fundamentally, disabled individuals were rarely stigmatized; instead, they were expected to share what gifts they had with the community."[12] The Indigenous Elders from different Nations I spoke with confirmed that their language had no word for disability, but admittedly there are a lot of languages and I was only able to speak to a few Elders.

A Look at the Statistics

In the article "Are We Handicapped, Disabled, or Something Else?' C. Edwin Vaughn explains that lexicographer John Simpson reaserched the word "disability" and traced the root word "ability" to France in the Middle Ages. "Disability, meaning a lack of ability to do something, took until 1545 to come about. But it did not come from the French; the English came up with it.[13]

Since disability means "not able," the question is: not able to do what?

American researchers Leslie Francis and Anita Silvers looked at how the term "disability" was first used in the legal sense, where disabled people were not recognized as individuals.[14] Disability then became a medical diagnosis, like we know it now.

Why are we as a society so fearful of the disability? I moved from going to the University of Alberta, where the campus is 800 acres (3.2 square kilometres), to going to a university whose campus was all in one building when I was 19. The second campus was smaller than a city block. I likely should have been using a walker, but I was scared of the way other people would look at me. I thought if there was a visible sign of disability, people would think of me as "lesser than." I am not sure how walking from wall to wall with an unsteady gait gave a better impression. I didn't tell anyone at the university about my multiple sclerosis until I first told the professor I had a crush on about my "defect." I knew I didn't have a chance with him (he married another student). Then I started using a manual wheelchair, which I figured was cool. Rick Hansen used a wheelchair, and he was amazing. A cane or a walker makes you look unfit, but a wheelchair can be captivating.

According to the MS Society of Canada, Canada has one of the highest rates of multiple sclerosis in the world, at about 1 in every 400 people.[15] The Society's Atlas of MS report found that, in Canada, almost 12 people are diagnosed with MS every day. The average age of diagnosis is 43 years, and 75% of the people living with MS are women. The majority, 90%, of people with MS are initially diagnosed with relapsing-remitting forms of MS, while 10% are diagnosed with progressive forms. In adherence with common practice, I was initially diagnosed with relapsing-remitting MS, but my neurologist said we had to wait and see how it developed. I have since re-classified myself as progressive MS, and my neurologist does not disagree.

Following the medical model, disabilities were initially broken down by diagnosis. Then all the disabilities were grouped together like one amorphous mass. All disabilities were equal. It didn't matter what your actual ability or lack of ability was, the fact that you had some kind of limitation was enough, for example, for the Ontarians with Disabilities Act. Now, we look to what we are trying to achieve. If there are any laws or campaigns, they no longer refer to disability but instead look to the end goal, whether it be inclusion or accessibility, such as is laid out in Accessible Nova Scotia.

In Canada, more than six million Canadians — 22% of the over-15 population — report having one or more disabilities that limit them in their daily activities. That is more than one in five. Your likelihood of having a disability increases with age, from 13% for those aged 15 to 24 years to 47% for those aged 75 and over, with women more likely to have a disability than men. Most individuals with a disability don't work because they can't. The majority would love a job, but their disability limits them. I would love to have employment, but my lack of voice makes that not feasible. Not surprisingly, the rate of employment for people with disabilities is lower than for people without disabilities. People with disabilities aged 25 to 64 years are less likely to be employed (only 59% have a job) compared to those without disabilities (80% are employed). Disabilities related to pain, flexibility, mobility and mental health were the most common types.[16] That's why it is crucial that disability supports pay above the poverty line.

In Nova Scotia — where I live — we get another story. The rates are much higher here; 30.4% aged 15 and older have at least one disability; with women being slightly more represented. The rate for youth aged 15–24 is 21%; and 29% of working-age adults (25–64) and 41% of older adults (65+) in Nova Scotia have at least one disability. In Nova Scotia, they do not ask whether you have a disability or not. Instead, they ask how many disabilities you have. The four most common disability types in Nova Scotia are related to pain (19.8%), flexibility (14.2%), mobility (13.3%) and mental health (11.8%). Other disability types are related to dexterity (6.7%), hearing (6.6%), seeing (6.6%), memory (5.3%), learning (5.3%) and development (1.3%).[17]

All the stats about disability seem to be employment focused. Is that the main feature of ability? That seems to be what is most important. It makes me wonder why that is most important to government. Is it because income tax on employment is the main source of revenue for the feds? Is that how we as people should look at the value of each hour? My assistant commented that they have worked a lot of jobs which could be done sitting down but the employer prefers them to be standing up. Employers think it looks more "professional" to be upright. This requirement eliminates a lot of people from the possibility of working those jobs. Someone with impaired flexibility or pain issues may not be able to stand for an entire shift, but if they were able to sit for part of the time they could be employed.

The father of one of my assistants had polio as a child. He would not dream of calling himself disabled even though he has difficulty with walking and balance. Disability seems to be a hated word among people of a certain generation. I believe that it comes from the view that having a disability means that you are less than, that you are not a whole person.

Ableism

Why is our society so ableist? If we are able-bodied, it is temporary. I suspect that most people don't realize the fleeting nature of their abilities. They think they will always have them. You don't need to be disabled to experience ableism. Maybe I learned early. My multiple sclerosis became apparent when I was only 15. I didn't have a chance to be oblivious to how temporary my status as able-bodied was. I don't think many people have the privilege of becoming disabled early in life; a lot of people seem to think you are either born with a disability or get to live your life free of it until you are "old." But disability is persistent, and it lurks around every corner.

When I went to the University of King's College in Halifax for journalism, they were doing some work on the exterior of the arts and administration building. Most people would just walk up the grand staircase at the front of the building. But for people who use wheelchairs, the entrance is at the back of the building. On the first day the director of the program was happy to help. But I couldn't ask for his help every time I wanted to enter the building. This meant on other days while the construction was going on I had to find a worker who was willing to carry my wheelchair over the worksite. I was lucky to find accommodating staff. I was able to manage the worksite on my own for the rest of the period they were working. The restoration crew was simply unaware of my needs.

When does it stop being the responsibility of individuals with a disability to make sure things are accessible, and when does society realize that accessibility is a problem for everyone?

A definition of ableism I borrowed from the Disability Filibuster conference on May 6, 2022, understands ableism as "a system of assigning value to people's bodies and minds based on societally constructed ideas of normalcy, productivity, desirability, intelligence, excellence, and fitness."[18] The socially constructed part is important.

I am currently watching *Love on the Spectrum* on Netflix. It is a wonderful reminder of how varied our abilities and outlooks are even if they are different by only a matter of degree. The people on the show, who are on the autistic spectrum, are not that different from me. That may not always appear to be the case. I know people who are autistic who are nonverbal and who are destructive to themselves and their caregivers. However, it may not be the autism that makes them destructive but the lack of the means to communicate their needs. It reminds us how ableism creates a divide in value based on our differences.

If people with disabilities are truly going to be integrated into the community, then there will be increased competition between the abled-bodied and the disabled. Contrary to what society seems to assume, the able-bodied will not always come out on top. When I wrote my first book I was in a competition for the Margaret and

John Savage First Book Award for Non-fiction. I was competing against two able-bodied authors, one of whom I was with in the Master of Fine Arts program at the University of King's College. She was amazing. I won the award. I wonder how the others felt losing to a person with a disability, or if they even recognized me as a person with a disability. I did also wonder if the fact that I won was merely because I have a disability.

In *Living Gently in a Violent World*, authors Jean Vanier and Stanley Hauerwas say, "But as we live with people who have been crushed, as we begin to welcome the stranger, we will gradually discover the stranger inside of us."[19] To me, what the authors are saying is that society does not easily accommodate differences. "The system" does not deal well with outsiders. If we spend more time with people with disability, we will all realize that not everything within us is as perfect as we would like to believe. Society is structured in such a way as to try to keep people with disability away from the able-bodied. We see them as two different categories, but in reality, even the individual with a flawless façade has broken parts. The authors add, "The danger is what Martin Luther King Jr. said: we have this tendency to push some people down so that we can rise up." I interpret this as the people who tend to be pushed down are the people with disabilities.

Ian Brown talks about a similar thing in his book *Boy in the Moon: A Father's Search for His Disabled Son*. He says, "Because in a competitive world, you must hide what is weak or wrong. Someone will try to beat you when they discover a weakness, try to take advantage of the weakness… And that is exactly where the [disabled] disagree. They respect our mutual weakness."[20]

People with disabilities need to be more self-assured because everyone else assumes that we cannot do it, or at least cannot do it as well as an able-bodied person can. The "it" can be work,[21] relationships, anything really. But the evidence does not lie: the accomplishments of people with disabilities should prove to society that people with disabilities can. We can.

Identity and Language

The saying goes, a rose by any other name would smell as sweet. The same is not true for people with disabilities.

I prefer tulips to roses but that's neither here nor there. Actually, when the man I moved to Nova Scotia to be with bought me roses for my birthday, I was a bit offended. Had he not been listening to anything I said? Maybe that was harsh, or maybe it was a sign.

When I was hired as the director of the Nova Scotia League for Equal Opportunities, I was pretty green. At the time you could be forgiven for most mistakes you made unless you failed to use person-first language. It meant identifying someone as a person before identifying them with a particular condition.

In my spare time I am the Atlantic representative on the Writers' Union of Canada. I was shocked the other day when I received an email from an individual who doesn't believe in the person-first approach. They were an adherent of the identity-first approach. I understand why the individual feels that their disability fundamentally changes who they are. If you are deaf, you cannot interact with the hearing world without an interpreter. The article "Person First and Identity First Language" states, "It is important to note that while person first language is often used in more formal writing, many people with disabilities, particularly younger people, are choosing to use identity first language."[22]

I am old. I like the person-first language approach. I do not want to be called multiple sclerosis even if the words champion or survivor are also attached. In this book, I use both approaches.

How do you evaluate one disability against another? Who can say which disability is worse and according to what criterion? Would you rather be blind or deaf? Would you rather be a quadriplegic or have autism? They are impossible questions and there is no right answer. Having a disability colours the way we interact with the world. We cannot answer with any degree of autonomy. Our perceptions are entirely a product of our backgrounds and our experiences.

I think a person with a disability is all-consumed by that condition. I am not saying that the individual is all-consumed by their particular ailment, but it colours the way they experience the world. If the individual has more than one condition, I think they both compete for airspace within the individual's mind. I am speculating because I only have one diagnosis at the moment, but when I had an eating disorder it lived quite comfortably alongside my multiple sclerosis. Certain parts of my disability require different skills. I find that spelling with my eyes requires a lot of patience. Not only from me but from the individual who is helping me with partner assisted scanning.

Medical Assistance in Dying (MAID) Legislation

I remember discussing the Sue Rodriguez case in my grade 10 social studies class. Rodriguez was a woman from British Columbia with amyotrophic lateral sclerosis (ALS) who wanted to be able to end her life when she saw fit. The Supreme Court of Canada ruled against her in a five to four decision. Why was it illegal for Rodriguez to hasten her inevitable death?

That was in 1993. In June 2016, terminally ill Canadians got the right to pursue medical assistance in dying (MAID) with the passage of Bill C-714: An Act to amend the Criminal Code. This means that if you have a terminal condition, you are entitled to end your life. With this legislation, Canada finally caught up to some of its European counterparts. In Switzerland, medically assisted suicide has been legal since 1942; in the Netherlands, since 2002. Before, there were a lot of attempted suicides by securing a plastic bag over one's head or trying to die by carbon monoxide poisoning.

A 2020 report from Justice Canada reads, "On September 11, 2019, the Superior Court of Québec found that it was unconstitutional to limit access to MAID to people nearing the end of life."[23] Subsequently, in 2021, the MAID law was amended to include all people with disabilities, whether their condition was terminal or not.

This sent the message to the disabled community that it is more appropriate if they are dead than alive. David Onley, former lieutenant-governor of Ontario, who uses a powerchair and has long advocated for governments to make policies that benefit people with disabilities, says it would be more accurate to call MAID "physician-assisted suicide." The bill, he says, would "make it easier for a person who is desperately entrapped, just barely holding on mentally and emotionally because of lack of government assistance, and psychologically beaten up because the system does not provide the support that it should provide — that they go to their doctor and say, 'I can't cope anymore.'"[24] Their physician can write a prescription for a lethal amount of medication.

As a cynic, I think the Bill C-7 amendments are the government's way of advocating for people with disabilities to off themselves. People with disabilities are expensive and demand a lot financially from government. They also do not usually generate a lot of revenue for government coffers.

At a session hosted by the Disability Filibuster on ableism on May 6, 2022, it was said that "80% of doctors assume that disability equates with suffering." Similarly, in her book *Too Late to Die Young*, Harriet McBryde Johnson writes, "They all assumed the only answers were prevention and cure."[25] This is not true unless you use a broad and all-encompassing definition of suffering. I am a quadriplegic due to my progressive multiple sclerosis. I cannot walk or be heard very well. Yet, I laugh and love. I do not think of myself as suffering. But if the learned community of medical professionals understands my life as one of suffering, it is no wonder that the politicians in Ottawa passed the expansion to Bill C-7.

It is entirely understandable why the disability movement has adopted the catch phrase "Nothing about us, without us." If the advice that the medical community is giving the government is that all people with disabilities are suffering, no wonder the federal government expanded the MAID legislation. But having a disability does not mean you are suffering. When I was capable of working, I did. Even now I earn what I can. It is not extravagant, but I do not have to eat only what is on sale at the grocery store. It is the lack of supports that leads to suffering. As a panelist said in the disability and poverty webinar held on June 24, 2022, by the Disability Filibuster, "Poverty is a policy decision."[26]

So, the government should not have been rushing to write new legislation making it easier for people with disabilities to kill themselves. What they should be doing is providing more support for people with disabilities. The disability amount you get with the Canadian Pension Plan should be above the poverty line. If you are on income assistance because of your disability, you should be over the poverty line. The poverty that is endemic to people with disabilities is the fault of government decision-making.[27] Less than 500,000 people with disabilities were getting CPP disability benefits in 2017, with a total payout from the federal government of $4.4 billion.[28] The government still had enough money to buy a pipeline at a cost of about $12 billion for the oilsands despite warnings from climate scientists.[29]

All the people who will be living in the units of the Shared Attendant Program are people with disabilities. They all could commit suicide under the recently enacted legislation, but I hope that their quality of life will only increase with the program.

At a webinar held by the Disability Filibuster on May 20, 2022, there was a lot of discussion about whether minors with a disability that are not terminally ill should be offered MAID.[30] The consensus was no, for all the above reasons. The right of a mature minor to have MAID is still up in the air, and there's a lot of discussion about it.[31] But there are also calls to extend the law to minors over 12 years of age who have a grievous and irremediable medical condition.

To me, that is understandable. It is only when there are no restrictions on the type and extent of disability that I have a problem with medical assistance in dying. A lot of participants in the web conference reflected on their own past and knew that if they had had the option of ending it all, they likely wouldn't be here. Our lives are innumerably better that they did not have the option of medical assistance in dying just because society may have made them suffer.

Many distinguished and amazing people have disabilities. The 16th president of the United States, Abraham Lincoln, lived with a tendency to become depressed that was often debilitating. It is surmised that he had Marfan syndrome, a condition of the connective tissue (there weren't the medical tests to diagnose Marfan in the 19th century). Ray Charles, who went blind at age seven due to glaucoma, was a celebrated pianist who developed his skills at a school for the blind. He mixed his talent for classical piano, which was all he could play at school, with his love for gospel and blues to create soul music. Robin Williams committed suicide after a diagnosis of Parkinson's disease. Prior to that, the legend of film had dealt with attention deficit hyperactive disorder and a bipolar diagnosis. An obvious figure with a disability was Stephen Hawking, who was diagnosed with ALS when he was 21, but what he did is beyond most of us. He made theoretical physics accessible to the average individual in his 1988 book, *A Brief History of Time: From the Big Bang to Black Holes.*

We need to remember that having a disability need not be a death sentence.

What I Will and Won't Miss

The current Self-Managed Care Program delivered by the Department of Health and Wellness has both positive aspects and elements that are hard to cope with. When we move from the system that provides only six or seven hours of attendant care per day to the Shared Attendant Program, there will be a lot of change. Things will be different. No longer will homecare be provided on a one-to-one basis. Though the individual will receive one-to-one care, there will be other participants in the unit receiving care from that same attendant.

I won't miss trying to fill in shifts when someone calls in sick. With Self-Managed Care, you are the program administrator, and it is your responsibility to fill in any program gaps. I know that illnesses are unavoidable and no one wants to be sick, but it throws a huge kink in my carefully planned schedule. This spring was challenging. I got a phone call from Spencer House (a local seniors' centre) reporting that someone had tested positive for COVID-19. As I had been at Spencer House for a toenail care appointment with my assistants Emily and Rae, we were all at risk. Rae came down with COVID-19. That meant I had to cancel their shifts for the next seven days. (Rae had two vaccine shots and a booster so they were only required to isolate for a week.) However, it was Easter or Passover (depending on your religious affiliation) and four of my assistants were out of town or out of the country. On top of all that, it was the end of term so many of the students I hired had university final exams. It was not a good time for trying to find people to fill shifts.

I am not opposed to being alone for a while. However, Netflix has a habit of turning off if you cannot hit the keyboard, and

Google Chrome is much worse than Firefox for this. I am fine listening to the radio, and I am even okay with my own thoughts if that is the only option. However, I am worried about being alone in case of fire. I cannot independently evacuate, and I do not have a strong enough voice to yell for help. Even if a firefighter knocked on my door and opened it, I could not yell and inform them of my presence. I have been scared of fire since my stepbrother used to torment me with burning sticks when I was a little kid while we were camping. (It was not that he was irresponsible; he was sixteen and I was ten, so teasing was a natural instinct.) Though I know my building is well constructed, we have had two incidents where the fire trucks came to the building. My worry may not be well founded, but it is still a worry.

I can deal with the advertising for and hiring of new assistants, though I am happy not to do it. There have been times when I could not find an assistant to hire. I have gotten creative with where I advertise, but finding someone is often a matter of luck. My waning voice and my interesting way of speaking, because of my progressive MS, means that an assistant needs to be trained before they are ready to assist me. And I will not miss doing the paperwork for the assistants. My father, sister and brother-in-law are all public accountants, but I was not endowed with the accounting gene. I only took one accounting course in university and hated it. Record-keeping is not my strong suit.

Meeting new assistants and having the opportunity to interact with them one-on-one for eight or nine consecutive hours is something about the current model that I will miss. While hiring my own assistants can be a pain in the ass, it offers the wonderful experience of being able to meet new people who would otherwise never enter my life. Isaac and Farzan, my current personal assistants, began to talk about their childhoods and how they were treated. Unlike Farzan, who had to deal with hand-me-down toys and trucks from his two older brothers, Isaac talked about his sister and how he always had toys but was more interested in books. I have had international students from Iran, Nigeria, Jamaica, Trinidad and Tobago, Zimbabwe, India, Kenya, Bangladesh and St. Lucia. I would never otherwise encounter such a breadth of experience. All my assistants seem to share a great respect for their parents.

I gave control of the administration of the four-person pilot to Independent Living Nova Scotia. I thought this made a better proposal, but giving up power is not something that comes naturally for me. I am a control freak. I know this and freely admit it. It leads me to a lot of wondering. How are the people in the program going to have a say over who is hired?

I know I was the one who put in the proposal to the Department of Community Services, but I don't think I ever worked out what the Shared Attendant Program would be like for me personally. I was lost in the glow of the fact that it will be getting three people younger than me out of nursing homes. When I go to sleep with Tom's weight next to me, I don't want to think about what it will be like in the Shared Attendant Program.

However, when Tom's blood sugar is low and he is passed out on the floor and I am alone and unable to call the paramedics, I will be singing a different tune. The situation has only gotten worse. I do not think it is fair for me to expect Tom when his blood sugar is low to read my lips or engage in partner-assisted scanning. Thankfully, Tom understands my whisper when I say "get juice." If I think about it, I will be very happy to have the attendants who can offer Tom juice, but right now, it feels more complicated than it ought to be. I need to work out a system where the attendants will know when to check on Tom and when to leave us alone.

As I get older, I wonder how much the way things were can continue into the future. I used to think of myself as an older sister to my assistants. But with the last assistant I hired, I realized I am the same age as his mother. I am no longer the wise older sister. I am the mother who nags. Maybe I am beyond the age of hiring students.

Accommodation

The Nova Scotia provincial government is serious about becoming accessible. The government is willing to accommodate your needs, but what if you don't know what your needs are?

If you are born with your disability, you have ample time to learn how you need things to be done, but if you have a progressive condition like I have, your changing needs are more difficult to nail down. You simply don't know how to accommodate yourself, what to ask for.

I used to be understood when I talked. That changed. I knew people needed to learn my voice, so I worked that into how I train new assistants. Then I lost my voice entirely as I was nearing the completion of the manuscript for this book. My older sister thought it was a great way to use the final gasps of my voice. She thought what could be more memorable than writing a work of non-fiction. She was coming to Halifax to visit from her home in Alberta. I thought it might put a kink in her holiday plans. Luckily, she just rolled with it. Her daughter had had a hard time with learning, and being a parent has really changed my sister. While she is still the same older sister that I grew up with, she has matured and developed a new side of herself. It has really changed her perspective on the world.

I had applied for a part-time position as a senior policy analyst with the Office of Accessibility. I did not get the job, but the process taught me a lot about how to ask for accommodations. At the time, I knew I was perfect for the position, but I had only lost my voice a few weeks earlier. I didn't know how to accommodate my new disability. I didn't know what to ask for or what accommodations employers would be willing to give.

I had a post-interview meeting with the woman who had interviewed me. She would have gladly accommodated my needs, but I didn't know what my needs were. I had asked for extra time to write down my answers, but I had only asked for a few hours. I soon realized that I needed more like a couple of days, not a few hours. But the lack-of-voice disability was new to me. How could I know what to ask for and how would the employer react to my request? I know by law people with disabilities are to be accommodated, but how far does that go? The woman I talked to was willing to do whatever I needed, but I didn't know what I needed. A few months later I know how long it takes me to type a couple of thousand words.

The Need for Group Homes in Nova Scotia

King's Meadow, the first group home in Nova Scotia, opened in 1969 in the community of Windsor.[32] It was a joint venture between the Canadian Progress Club of Halifax and the Canadian Association of Community Living. It is a place for people with intellectual disabilities.

One must ask why people with intellectual disabilities were treated differently than people with severe physical disabilities. Maybe people with intellectual disabilities are not a medical problem that needs to be solved.

As mentioned earlier, the 1986 book *The Principle of Normalization in Human Services* by Wolf Wolfensberger details how people with disabilities should be given every opportunity to live like the general population. He was usually referring specifically to individuals with intellectual disabilities, but he doesn't always specify that group. To me the author is recognizing that all individuals with disabilities need the opportunity to live lives just like other people do.

The Shared Attendant Program that we proposed to the Department of Community Services does just that. It gives people with severe physical disabilities the opportunity to live like everyone else. My partner can stay overnight if he wants to. My mother can come for a visit. I can own two cats if they don't eat each other alive. Rather than being placed in a nursing home, people who need 24-hour care can get that while still living within the community.

Wendy Lill is a former MP for Dartmouth–Cole Harbour. She is the chair of Community Homes Action Group, a playwright and the mother of a son with Down syndrome. In an interview I had with her, she wrote, "He was born in 1985, the year that persons with disabilities were recognized by the Charter of Rights and Freedoms as having rights under the Constitution. We took that very seriously and derived much hope from that." Lill continued:

> Advocacy and support groups such as Nova Scotia CAMR (Canadian Association for the Mentally Retarded) [which became the Canadian Association for Community Living and is now Inclusion Canada] got parents together to talk about community-based supported living alternatives. Regional Residential Services Society really started from a group of parents who formed to start running some group homes. The federal government was very involved in the early years and worked with municipalities and provided substantial funding initially to get community options happening.

The Canada Assistance Plan, an effort by the Canadian government to help provinces deal with healthcare and social assistance costs, funded a number of group homes. The program has since ended.

Under the division of powers between the federal government and the provinces, the province is responsible for social and community services. The federal government should not be involved. In 1996, the province put a moratorium on the building of all new group homes. Wendy Lill says the idea was for the province to "catch its breath."

Nova Scotians with disabilities have been waiting for a plan from government for a long time. In June 2013, while part of the Nova Scotia Joint Community–Government Advisory Committee on Transforming the Services to Persons with Disabilities (SPD) Program, Wendy Lill and Lynn Harwell co-wrote *Choice, Equality and Good Lives in Inclusive Communities: A Roadmap for Transforming the Nova Scotia Services to Persons with Disabilities Program*.[33] According to the Disability Rights Coalition, "Contrary to its commitment to the *Roadmap* in October of 2013, the Nova Scotia government through its Disability Supports Program, is assisting fewer people with disabilities in 2021 than in 2013, when it committed to the *Roadmap*, dropping from 5,184 to 5,033 people." Institutionalizing people with disabilities fell out of favour with the world in the 1970s. "Nova Scotia is the last province in Canada to rely on these institutions," says the Disability Rights Coalition. The Coalition also says, "Numbers supplied to the Coalition by the Department of Community Services show the waitlist [for group homes] has grown from 1,099 in 2014 to 1,915 in 2021, an increase of 74%."[34]

The Department of Community Services in Nova Scotia now says that all disabilities are equal and that all disabilities need to be handled with the same care and concern. As mentioned earlier, this was not always the case. People with intellectual disabilities were granted their own small option homes in the 1970s after extensive work by the parents and caregivers, confirms Wendy Lill.

In spite of half a century of community living, people with intellectual disabilities are not as worthy as their non-disabled counterparts. They are tolerated, not included. I think tolerance is a more apt description than inclusion because it seems that people with intellectual disabilities are not really part of the community. They are simply tolerated. That must be a hard way to live — to know that the community doesn't really want you but merely puts up with your presence.

"The physical disability substantially limits functional independence and results in the person requiring ongoing support and skill development," says the Department of Community Services.[35] I agree with the first part but not the second. Why do we need skill development? I think everyone needs skill development. The severely physically disabled people do not need it more than anyone else. It is disheartening to hear that a group of educated individuals at Community Services think that skill development would help those with severe physical disabilities. I do not think that any amount of training will give me the use of my legs or hands back.

Bill 59

Canada adopted the Accessible Canada Act in 2010, although Ontario beat the feds to the punch, having adopted the Accessibility for Ontarians with Disabilities Act in 2005. Manitoba followed the national government, adopting the Accessibility for Manitobans Act in 2013. On September 18, 2017, Nova Scotia followed suit, adopting Bill 59, also known as the Accessibility Act. With it, Nova Scotia vowed to become accessible to people with all types of disabilities by 2030.

Why Nova Scotia wants to adopt accessibility legislation makes sense — the province is at the top of the mountain when it comes to disability rates. According to novascotia.ca, 30% of Nova Scotians aged 15 years and older have at least one disability. The Canadian average is 22.3%.[36] Kevin Murphy, a quadriplegic and former speaker of the Nova Scotia House of Assembly, was quoted in a document leading up to "Public Input to Shape Accessibility

Legislation" as saying, "Nova Scotians with disabilities want to participate in work and education, family and community life, and to be a vibrant part of the great Province we call home."[37]

Former MLA and now political commentator Graham Steele explained in a CBC article entitled "Upcoming public hearings a change from 'ridiculously unfriendly' norm" that "a legislative committee will resume public hearings on Bill 59, the Accessibility Act. The hearings will be a model of citizen-centered public engagement, which will be a sharp contrast to the usual, perfunctory, MLA-centred public hearings."[38]

The Law Amendments Committee is usually just something that needs to be done. It is a box to check. All governments in Canada need to give the public a chance to comment on legislation before it becomes law. But most law amendments are merely for show. The government personnel are not usually there because they want to be, but because they have an obligation to be. The amendments for Bill 59 were not like that. They were more substantial. The Bill 59 Community Alliance worked to get the Bill redrafted.[39] It happened. The government rewrote the Bill according to the principles laid out by the Community Alliance. The law amendments occurred when the House was not sitting so there was no strict schedule. The amendments sessions were held in the morning, afternoon and evening. They had sign language interpreters, captioning available, sighted interpreters and the like. The government of Nova Scotia was going to get it right.

Gerry Post, a former leader with the Bill 59 Community Alliance who went on to become the first ever executive director of the Accessibility Directorate of Nova Scotia, told me that the Community Alliance had 37 organizations having to do with persons with disabilities and accessibility sign off on the principles developed for the second round of the Law Amendments Committee.

When I heard about the province's goal of becoming accessible by 2030, I laughed. Nova Scotia still puts people with severe physical disabilities in nursing homes. When I talked to my mother about having people with severe physical disabilities living in the community, she said, "I think your community living idea is a much-needed housing alternative for younger/mid-aged adults with severe physical disabilities. It promotes positive emotional and intellectual health while providing required physical care. It fosters community inclusion and acceptance of individuals with differing physical abilities. Healthy alternatives to institutional long-term care are long overdue."

The province has an action plan to help more Nova Scotians with disabilities work and live as independently as possible in their community. If the province truly wants a place where people can live, it must work to help make that a reality.

Province Stalls Prototype Home for Disabled Young Adults on Gottingen

(*Opinion editorial submitted to the* Halifax Examiner *in November 2019 by Jen Powley*)

After the 2019 Emerald Hall decision affirmed that people with disabilities have the right to adequate care in the community. And after the UN Special Rapporteur on the Rights of Persons with Disabilities gave a scathing report on how Nova Scotia is doing on housing in her preliminary comments (Nova Scotia still has over 1000 people in institutions and a waitlist of over 1,500 for group homes), you would think that the government of Nova Scotia would jump at the chance to give people with severe physical disabilities a home within the community, but that doesn't appear to be the case.

Though the Nova Scotia government ended the moratorium on the building of new group homes (though 400 group homes are needed, not just the two announced.) And though the government has enough sense to put the Accessibility Directorate under the Department of Justice. And though the government has passed the Accessibility by Design Act saying that the province will be fully accessible by 2030.

Nine months after Independent Living Nova Scotia, EcoGreen Homes and I presented a proposal to the Department of Community Services that would give me and three other young adults the option of staying out of a nursing home through shared attendant care at little more than the cost of keeping us in a nursing home, we still haven't had an answer from the department on whether the developer can move ahead on the proposal. The developer has left the space on Gottingen Street untouched at great expense to himself. After the presentation, the developer was asked how long the province had to get back to him. He answered, three months.

We haven't hand-picked the other three young people. We had hoped Joanne Larade, who had worked on doing research with the Schulich School of Law at Dalhousie University, could be one of the residents. Larade was a disability rights activist with Muscular Dystrophy Canada, Independence Now, and Empowered. She has passed away since the project was proposed. Larade joined No More Warehousing, convinced people with severe physical disabilities could together do something to fight for the dignity we deserve in housing. Like other Nova Scotians, we deserve choice in where and how we each live and with whom.

Unfortunately, she passed away while the government dragged its heels. We are allowing the government a chance to decide which three young people it would be best to give a chance to be a real part of the community rather than living on the outskirts. We are hoping that in the future no young people will be put in nursing homes and that our unit will be a prototype. We don't believe keeping people under 60 in a nursing home where most people are in a different stage of their lives is good for the mental health of the young people. Just because a 90-year-old needs physical assistance doesn't mean they should be lumped together with a young person who needs the same level of care.

We would like the Government of Nova Scotia to approve the proposal we presented to them on February 28. We would like to see EcoGreen Homes get the go-ahead. We would like Independent Living Nova Scotia to be involved in developing a home for people with severe physical disabilities.

A Glacial Pace

The developer, Edward Edelstein, was explicit when we met with the Department of Community Services. He could reserve the first floor of the building he was developing on Gottingen Street in Halifax's North End for three months. After that, Edelstein had to move on to other offers. He couldn't guarantee the space for the Shared Attendant Program pilot.

As the time from when we presented our proposal to the Department of Community Services grew longer, Edelstein became increasingly unsettled. He really liked the idea of developing a home in the community for adults with severe physical disabilities. Before he was a developer, he taught biology and woodworking with the Waldorf school. In the Waldorf school movement, everything that is done aims to "nurture the healthy, holistic development of each individual child."[40]

Edelstein designed a project for Camphill Communities Ontario, including a building and trails at their group farm, converting a barn into an office and renovating a group home. Considering the needs of people with disabilities was not new to him. He lent me the 2010 book *The Sound of a Wild Snail Eating*. Written by Elisabeth Tova Bailey, it explores the relationship between bedridden Bailey and a wild snail that has taken up residence on her nightstand. The book explores themes of wonder and confinement. I thought it was an apt story for an individual whose multiple sclerosis changes the way she interacts with society.

I am constantly amazed by how well-versed Canadian society is on accessibility needs. *Maybe* the province's idea of an accessible Nova Scotia by 2030 isn't impossible. Edelstein was willing to design the space to my exact specifications. He got his own design team to develop a plan just as I desired at his own expense. But Edelstein became very frustrated working with the province. He saw them as "refusing to choose who could live in the space." He saw us as having "a space, and a certified caregiver organization." The province would not agree to fund it until 11 months after the initial presentation. Even a few days before we got an official word from the province, Edelstein was trying to change the way we were getting participants. He said in an email, "If you get the three others who want to live on Gottingen Street, then think about going public with that. That way it would be difficult for the government to back out. It sure seems fishy to me that they took our project out of their approval."

Edelstein wanted us to advertise for participants and do the selection outside of government plans. We were never really in control of participant selection. The letters about the program that offered 24-hour support were sent from the Department of Health and Wellness, not from ILNS. If we tried to hurry government, they would probably just take longer. Edelstein's idea might get us three people with severe physical disabilities, but it would do nothing to build a relationship with the Department.

Edelstein was not familiar with the glacial pace of the provincial government. Both Carrie and I had worked with government long enough — Carrie (with ILNS) and myself (as a sustainable transportation coordinator at the Ecology Action Centre) — to know that the pace was glacial. Eventually we decided to release Edelstein from any moral obligations he felt towards the project. We couldn't guarantee him any movement, and it was not fair to hold him back from doing what he needed to do. He had been a great supporter of what we were trying to accomplish. His idea to advertise for people with disabilities was great, but we knew that it would be jumping the queue. People living in nursing homes deserved a chance to relocate into the community, and his idea depended on the individual having friends or family see the advertisement and contact the appropriate people.

Carrie and I knew government had to work through their own processes. We decided to send an email to Edelstein breaking off the relationship. He thought like a developer and hoped that the rest of us would operate on a similar schedule. Unfortunately, it was only a few days later that I got an email from the Department of Community Services asking if I would have a phone date with Kelly Regan, then minister of Department of Community Services. Carrie assumed it was good news. I reserved judgement, knowing I would be crushed if the proposal got this far and then was rejected. I didn't want to set up false expectations.

In January of 2020, a full 11 months after we had proposed the project to the Department of Community Services, I called Kelly Regan's office. I was a few minutes late for the call. I have an analogue clock on my wall and I guess it was set wrong. I am legally blind and cannot read a digital clock. Carrie was also on the call. She was right — I had nothing to worry about. Regan announced that the project had been approved; it was going to happen. Now we just needed to figure out how.

Notes

1. Harriet McBryde Johnson, *Too Late to Die Young* (New York: Picador, 2006), 203.
2. Harriet McBryde Johnson, 179.
3. Government of Canada, "Disability Tax Credit," June 24, 2022. canada.ca/en/revenue-agency/services/tax/individuals/segments/tax-credits-deductions-persons-disabilities/disability-tax-credit.html.
4. Michael Oliver, *The Politics of Disablement* (Palgrave Macmillan, 1990).
5. Centers for Disease Control and Prevention, "Disability and Health Overview," September 16, 2020. https://www.cdc.gov/ncbddd/disabilityandhealth/disability.html.
6. Z. Swaine, "Medical Model," in *Encyclopedia of Clinical Neuropsychology*, edited by J.S. Kreutzer, J. DeLuca, and B. Caplan (New York, Springer, 2011). https://doi.org/10.1007/978-0-387-79948-3_2131.
7. Rosecrest Communities, "Eden Alternative: Eden Principles of Care," n.d. rosecrest.ca/facilities/facilities-sagewood/facilities-sagewood-eden.
8. Simi Linton, "Reassigning Meaning," in *The Disability Studies Reader*, edited by Davis J. Lennard (New York: Routledge, 2006), p.162.

9. Linton, "Reassigning Meaning," p. 163.

10. Roy F. Baumeister, "Effects of Social Exclusion and Interpersonal Rejection: An Overview with Implications for Human Disability," in *The Paradox of Disability: Responses to Jean Vanier and L'Arche Communities from Theology and the Sciences,* edited by Hans S. Reinders (Wm. B. Eerdmans Publishing, 2010): 51–59.

11. Nicole Ineese-Nash, "Disability as a Colonial Construct: The Missing Discourse of Culture in Conceptualizations of Disabled Indigenous Children," *Canadian Journal of Disability Studies,* 9, 3 (2020). https://cjds.uwaterloo.ca/index.php/cjds/article/view/645.

12. Dustin Galer, *Work Disability in Canada: Portraits of a System* (Lulu Press, 2017).

13. Edwin Vaughn, "Are We Handicapped, Disabled, or Something Else?" *Braille Monitor*, January 2019. nfb.org//sites/default/files/images/nfb/publications/bm/bm19/bm1901/bm190111.htm.

14. Leslie Francis and Anita Silvers, "Perspectives on the Meaning of Disability," *AMA Journal of Ethics,* 18, 10: 1025–1033 (2016). https://journalofethics.ama-assn.org/article/perspectives-meaning-disability/2016-10.

15. MS Society of Canada, "Prevalence and Incidence of MS in Canada and Around the World," December 20, 2020. mssociety.ca/research-news/article/prevalence-and-incidence-of-ms-in-canada-and-around-the-world.

16. Statistics Canada, *Canadian Survey on Disability, 2017*, November 28, 2018. www150.statcan.gc.ca/n1/daily-quotidien/181128/dq181128a-eng.htm. For more information and other reports, see Statistics Canada's "Reports on Disability and Accessibility in Canada." www150.statcan.gc.ca/n1/en/catalogue/89-654-X.

17. Government of Nova Scotia, "Prevalence of Disabilities in Nova Scotia," n.d. novascotia.ca/accessibility/prevalence.

18. Disability Filibuster, "Everyday Ableism = Dehumanized Every Day" (webcast), May 6, 2022. disabilityfilibuster.ca.

19. Stanley Hauerwas and Jean Vanier, *Living Gently in a Violent World: The Prophetic Witness of Weakness* (Inter-varsity Press, 2008), p. 70.

20. Ian Brown, *Boy in the Moon: A Father's Search for His Disabled Son* (Toronto: Random House of Canada, 2010), p. 232.

21. Government of Canada, *Rethinking DisAbility in the Private Sector*, April 27, 2022. https://www.canada.ca/en/employment-social-development/programs/disability/consultations/rethinking-disabilities.html

22. AskEARN. "Person First and Identity First Language," n.d. askearn.org/page/people-first-language.

23. Justice Canada, *What We Heard Report: A Public Consultation on Medical Assistance in Dying (MAID)*, April 2020. https://www.justice.gc.ca/eng/cj-jp/ad-am/wwh-cqnae/index.html.

24. Meagan Gillmore, "Catastrophic Pandora's Box': Disabled Ontarians Speak Out Against Proposed MAID Law," *TVO Today*, March 3, 2021. tvo.org/article/catastrophic-pandoras-box-disabled-ontarians-speak-out-against-proposed-maid-law.

25. Harriet McBryde Johnson, 50.

26. Disability Filibuster, "Disability and Poverty" (webcast), June 24, 2022. https://www.youtube.com/watch?v=k8J_VoVgeaY.

27. Katherine Wall, *Insights on Canadian Society: Low Income Among Persons with a Disability in Canada*, Statistics Canada, August 11, 2017. www150.statcan.gc.ca/n1/pub/75-006-x/2017001/article/54854-eng.htm.

28. Government of Canada, *Annual Report of the Canada Pension Plan for Fiscal Year 2017 to 2018*, April 21, 2022. canada.ca/en/employment-social-development/programs/pensions/reports/annual-2018.html.

29. Karin Kirk, "Canada's Oil Sands Industry Is Taking a Big Hit," Yale Climate Connections, March 5, 2021. yaleclimateconnections.org/2021/03/canadas-oil-sands-industry-is-taking-a-big-hit/.

30. Disability Filibuster, "Mature Minors and MAID Confirmation" (webcast), May 20, 2022. https://www.youtube.com/watch?v=6XymM0m93S8.

31. Dying with Dignity Canada, *Mature Minors and MAID: A Deep Dive into the Issues of the Parliamentary Review*, September 15, 2021. dyingwithdignity.ca/blog/pr_mature_minors/.

32. King's Meadow, "About us." https://kingsmeadow.wixsite.com/kmrs/about_us.

33. Wendy Lill and Lynn Hartwell, *Choice, Equality and Good Lives in Inclusive Communities: A Roadmap for Transforming the Nova Scotia Services to Persons with Disabilities Program*, Nova Scotia Joint Community-Government Advisory Committee on Transforming the Services to Persons with Disabilities (SPD) Program, June 2013.

34. Jennifer Henderson, "Report: Nova Scotia Failing to Meet Its Commitment to De-Institutionalize People with Disabilities," *Halifax Examiner*, July 20, 2021.

35. NS Department of Community Services, *Disability Support Program*, April 2022.

36. Province of Nova Scotia, "Disability in Nova Scotia." https://novascotia.ca/accessibility/stats-on-disability-in-Nova-Scotia.pdf.

37. Government of Nova Scotia, Dept. of Community Services, "Public Input to Shape Accessibility Legislation," press release, November 6, 2014. https://novascotia.ca/news/release/?id=20141106003.

38. Graham Steele, "Upcoming Public Hearings a Change from 'Ridiculously Unfriendly' Norm, says Graham Steele," *CBC News*, February 8, 2017. cbc.ca/news/canada/nova-scotia/graham-steele-public-hearings-blueprint-law-amendments-committee-1.3972290/.

39. The Bill 59 Community Alliance, "Principles to Redraft Bill 59, the Nova Scotia Accessibility Act," March 2, 2017. https:// nslegislature.ca/sites/default/files/pdfs/committees/62_3_ LACSubmissions/20170302/20170302-059-031.pdf.

40. South Shore Waldorf School, "About Us," n.d. waldorfns.org/ about-ssws/#about.

Chapter 3

THE ANSWER

Realization

Carrie Ernst, the executive director of Independent Living Nova Scotia (ILNS), does not think the Department of Health and Wellness in Nova Scotia was being malevolent towards people with disabilities by placing them in nursing homes; they simply did not have much imagination and did things exactly the way they had been done before. Erika Dyck in her article "Institutionalization" states, "The rise of institutions throughout the 1800s coincided with a social desire to isolate people in these facilities from mainstream society, often on a presumption of their danger to society."[1] The Department of Health and Wellness did not know how things could work any other way. They were firmly entrenched in the medical model of disability. They needed to think about disability in a new way. If they looked at disability from a social perspective that was developed by people with disabilities themselves rather than the medical model, they would see disability not as a thing to fix but as merely a way of being that is different than what is expected.

When ILNS was willing and able to do the research and consult on the administrative changes required, the province of Nova Scotia jumped at the opportunity, but it was a massive change. There were conflicting policies between the provincial government departments that all needed to be revamped.

But there were more problems. Nova Scotia seemed to be talking out of both sides of its mouth. On one side, it tried to appeal the decision on the Emerald Hall human rights case, but on April 14, 2022, the Supreme Court of Canada denied Nova Scotia the opportunity to appeal the provincial human rights decision. The attempt to appeal the human rights decision told people with disabilities that the province does not think it had acted inappropriately to begin with. On the other hand, the province is putting money into options for community living, which says that the community is where the litigants should have been living. Nova Scotia put in the 2022–23 budget that 200 non-seniors will be moved out of nursing homes over the following four years and into the community. What are people with disabilities to think?

The Department of Community Services has allowed the waitlist for group homes for people with intellectual disabilities to grow to nearly double. At the same time, they are embarking on the Shared Attendant Program. Are they really heartless, or are they just single-minded? Do they not realize that one is in opposition to the other?

They might be focusing on attendant care after they got a lot of negative press with one younger resident of the nursing home speaking out about what it was like to be in your 20s living with a group of seniors who were essentially waiting for death. I am not saying all older adults have lost the will to live, but when you are living with individuals with dementia it is hard to have a cheerful outlook. The individual who got the Department of Community Services all the press was Vicky Levack. Then there was our proposal. It was a perfect storm.

Independent Living

Carrie Ernst was working incessantly on the Shared Attendant Program and did not have time for any other duties of her position. She knew she would have to hire another person. Kathleen Odell's husband's family were all in Nova Scotia, and he used to spend summers on the South Shore. Carrie thought she might be able to convince Kathleen to move to the province. Carrie was a member of the board of Independent Living Canada and Kathleen was the chair. Carrie and Kathleen had become friends during their time together. They were out for dinner at the Upstreet BBQ Brewhouse in Dartmouth. (I have to assume the barbeque is more important to Carrie than the brewery, because when I asked about smells, the response I got focused on the amazing cornbread and the fabulous dipping sauces, not the beer.) Carrie brought up the idea of Kathleen applying for a position that had just become available with Inclusion Nova Scotia. Kathleen was willing to relocate from Toronto but didn't think the job was right for her. Then Carrie mentioned that she would be hiring a new person for the Shared Attendant Program. She didn't have the funding yet, but it would have to happen. She simply couldn't do all the work by herself, and it wasn't fair to expect her assistant to call developers. Kathleen was interested. She believes in the independent living philosophy.

With a mother and an aunt who were pioneers in the independent living movement, Kathleen couldn't help but be indoctrinated into their principles and philosophy. Kathleen grew up in a house that had been modified so that it was suitable for what her mother could do, for example, reach the light switches from her wheelchair. During her younger years Kathleen did not realize that society was not particularly disability friendly because everything her family did was only done if it was accessible. It wasn't until later in life that she realized that not everywhere was accommodating to wheelchairs.

When Kathleen was in grade primary, her mother insisted that Kathleen take her to school for "show and tell." Kathleen thought it was a little weird at the time, but her mother thought it was important for kids to have the opportunity to ask questions and see people with disabilities as part of the community.

Kathleen's mother made sure the school was accessible so that she could visit her daughter and attend events such as school plays. I asked Kathleen what it was like having a mother with a disability. Kathleen stressed that her mother was like any other mother. The only difference is that Kathleen had to bring the Band-Aid to her mother when she skinned her knee so that her mother could apply the bandage and kiss the wound better.

I don't want to give the idea that life was perfect for Kathleen. Once her mother tried to run her down with her wheelchair, and Kathleen had to jump on the couch for safety. But she also shared memories of watching *The Young and the Restless* with her mother when her mother was tired and had to lie down early. Kathleen's relationship with her mother is one of love, though she admits that she and her sister did not get along until they were in their early teens and must have driven their parents crazy before that.

When I interviewed Kathleen on June 2, 2022, she told me her philosophy is based on "the social model of disability. It is the model of disability that is in direct opposition to the medical model. And really the way that I would define independent living would be like the right to autonomy, the right to choose, the right to informed risk taking and the right to decision making and the right to be included in the community."

Kathleen told me that when she was pregnant, she had not worried that her daughter Sabrina would have spinal muscular atrophy even though it is hereditary. The mother and father both need to carry the genes for the condition. Also Kathleen's mother had invited Kathleen's family to live at her house if the baby did have the condition. The house was already fully accessible, so there was nothing to worry about. If the baby did have the condition, they would deal with it.

Kathleen was the obvious choice for working with Carrie. She was perfect for her role in helping to implement the shared services model. It was her birthday the day I interviewed her. When I asked what she wanted for her birthday, she replied, "I want the units off the ground up and running."

Kathleen inadvertently persuaded me that I was wrong to convince myself that I couldn't have kids. Maybe I couldn't hold a baby to my breast to feed, but it did not mean that I needed to dismiss the idea of parenthood so quickly. I know I would not be as laissez-faire about it as Kathleen, who didn't even mention her mother's spinal muscular atrophy to her obstetrician until she was in her second trimester. It wasn't that important to her. I, on the other hand, would have been clamouring for more information. I have multiple sclerosis, and the research about passing on the condition is not cut and dried. According to an article on the MS Society website, "Although multiple sclerosis is not strictly hereditary (directly transmitted from parent to child), the risk of developing MS is higher among siblings or children of a person with MS compared to the general population. This inheritance pattern suggests that genetic factors play a role in determining MS risk."[2] My father and my aunt both have multiple sclerosis. I am not as willing as Kathleen to subject my offspring to the condition.

The Medical Model versus the Independent Living Philosophy

There are basically two ways of looking at people who are not able-bodied. Earlier I discussed the medical model of care, which assumes that the individual is broken and needs medical treatment to make them whole again. The other way is understood through the independent living philosophy, which recognizes the individual as a complete person who may need help to achieve their goals but allows the individual to determine and direct their path.[3] If the medical model is at the heart of the problem of how we understand disability, then we should look at how the medical model came about.

The first thing we need to ask is the medical model of what? I think we are talking about the medical model of care. At the core is the thought that whatever problems exist can be alleviated with the use of medical techniques and knowledge; the model assumes there is a problem and that the problem is within the individual. "The origins of medicine are ambiguous, but all great ancient civilizations developed their own ways of healing the ill," says Giovanni Silvano.[4] In the Western World, the model we are most familiar with depends on Hippocrates and his four humours: yellow bile, black bile, blood and phlegm.[5] Silvano explains, "As postal services and other communications improved, medical knowledge was able to spread rapidly. Democracy led to people demanding health as a human right."

The independent living philosophy does not look to the individual as the start of all disability. Instead, it looks to the way society has developed. Unlike in the medical model, the social model of impairment assumes that the problem does not reside within the individual but in the social fabric that surrounds the individual. The problem is turned on its head. Independent living is about having choices, making decisions, taking risks, making mistakes and taking responsibility for your decisions.

I asked Carrie to be a part of the group home project way back in 2019. I didn't know how the Shared Attendant Program was going to work, but I like the independent living philosophy. I thought it needed a seat at our table. Kathleen was hired to be a point person for the independent living philosophy. She recounts in an email from June 30, 2022, "As a person who grew up and through the IL Philosophy with attendant services in my family home, my understanding is both deeply personal and nuanced. Before policy was designed or written there was a document to capture the philosophical approach for the shared attendant pilot for services from ILNS. The approach was that people with disabilities are the experts in their own lives and the services must be supportive with respect to individual differences and deeply respectful of the people accessing those services."

Carrie signs off her emails with the phrase, "ILNS champions the right to live independently and supports individuals in their pursuit of independence. It is the vision of ILNS that all Nova Scotians with disabilities have the ability to live a full, independent life at home, work, and play within an inclusive community." I thought the project needed a strong voice for people with disabilities. We all should hold to the ideals of self-determination. Carrie is that voice.

Buying the Unit Next Door

Maria, my neighbour, came to the door of my condo. Sometimes, Maria would share whatever she was baking, and I was hoping for warm tea biscuits or cookies fresh out of the oven. Instead, she had news that would rock my existence.

Maria had brought me gifts in the past. I had put my cat Tula down a couple of months before as she had cancer on her kidneys. Maria had brought me an electronic feline to cheer me up. It was black with tuxedo markings, and it meowed when you pet it and turned on its back so you could scratch its belly. It freaked out my partner. I kept it in the closet because Tom would mistake it for a real cat, and I gave it to my mother the next time she visited. In exchange we went to the SPCA in a neighbouring community and picked up two new cats (they were a bonded pair). Maria had cats of her own though one had recently disappeared. It went outdoors and never returned.

Maria announced that she was moving. Her husband had passed away a few months previously, on February 20, 2021. She thought paying condo fees when it was just her and the cats was ridiculous.

I had recently talked to Carrie about the problems she had been experiencing trying to find a home for the pilot. Carrie had gotten a lot of interest from building owners when she was initially talking to them about the Shared Attendant Program. But, with the vacancy rate in Halifax at less than 1%, any apartments that became available were snatched in record time. Why would a landlord leave a suite unoccupied while they waited for another unit on that floor to become available?

I thought that, with my unit and the unit next to mine, we would have enough room for the program. As soon as Maria left, I immediately went on the internet to find out what realtor Maria was working with because I wanted to get a realtor from the same firm. I thought there might be an advantage to having an agent with the same company. I don't know anything about how real estate really works but I have a fertile imagination. I would have to find someone with enough equity to buy Maria's unit. Carrie had talked about the program buying the unit eventually, but no board member in their right mind would vote to spend over $400,000 to buy a unit for a program that was still in the pilot stage.

I would have to turn to my family. I dialed my mother's number. She was not comfortable putting effort into a bid at that moment. She supported what I was thinking, but her mother was in the midst of a psychotic episode, and she couldn't deal with anything else (my grandmother was 97). I turned to my father. I hadn't lived with him since I was three, but he still was my father. Because he now uses a scooter due to his own progressive multiple sclerosis, he might be understanding of our predicament. He had given money to my sister, Candice, and her husband, in order for them to purchase their home. He gave my sister, Nicole, a vehicle to drive from her acreage to her contract work, wherever it might be. Nicole had become an accountant much to my father's delight. He saw her as carrying on his legacy. I thought asking him to buy the unit for the Shared Attendant Program was worth a shot. To my surprise and delight he said sure. I was a little leerier of the process than if my mother had been involved. With my mother, I can be certain that I am getting all the specifics. I knew that my mother would discuss all the details with me and would not make an offer without talking to me about it.

I told dad he could get a second mortgage on his house. He said there was no first mortgage so he could easily get one. My father recently sold his house on his farm and the land and equipment. His multiple sclerosis had advanced to make working on the farm equipment unsafe. He had to convert the shower in his own home to make it accessible. Everything I have recently learned about my father I learned second or third hand. It may be because I am over half the country away, or it might be because the only emails my father writes are cursory. My father is not the best communicator. It is my theory that this is what was at the heart of the marital breakdown (that and his habit of sleeping with other women; though that was not all bad because I got a great sister out of the deal). I have not seen my father in several years.

The real estate market in Halifax was super hot in 2021. A realtor named Mark Stein, with over three decades of experience, was featured on Global News claiming, "In my 32 years I've never experienced anything as — I don't want to say the word crazy — but anything as challenging as it is." Buyers might be paying nearly double the asking price. I thought my father should know that. I texted my real estate agent, Patti, to explain what we were trying to do. She thought what we were doing was a great idea, and she suggested that I write a letter to the woman selling the unit.

I introduced my father to Patti over a text. Things were out of my hands now. I had to wait. Patti called my father and told him that we were successful in getting the condo. I texted Carrie.

Carrie said that when she was notified of the purchase of the unit, she "cried... I had a couple of conversations with your dad. You know how when people say, I don't think thank you is enough, it just doesn't feel like it is enough. We were so deflated and had run into so many problems, trying to find suitable housing."

I am glad my father could help.

Closing

After we bought the unit, we had to take possession of the property. Because of my poor eyesight and because the unit was bought for ILNS, I thought Carrie and Kathleen should be at the closing. I asked Tom if he could be there too. We could use his long arms and his good eyesight for the inspection.

We all met the real estate agent in the lobby of the condo building. When Patti entered the condo, she immediately turned on all the taps and flipped on the stove burners and the oven. She wanted to make sure everything was in working order. She had obviously done this before.

I wasn't prepared for the maelstrom of emotion that presented itself that morning. I should have brought tissues with me.

Carrie admits, "I cried that day that we did the closing. I have to tell you; I had no makeup left."

We were concerned about the ceiling in one of the bedrooms, which had obviously leaked at some point. It was dry so we assumed it was not a new or continuous problem. But we wanted it noted in the contract, so we were covered for liability. I didn't know how much of a stickler you had to be for details. Thankfully, both Carrie and Kathleen were tyrants of the deal.

When we were done with the inspection, we had to pose with the agent and the sold sign. People with disabilities in Canada often live in poverty. They typically earn less than do able-bodied people of the same gender and age. According to Easter Seals, men with disabilities typically earn $9,557 less than do able-bodied males of the same age; women earn $8,853 less.[6] Recent research confirms that "working-age Canadians with disabilities have employment rates that are almost 40 percent lower than the larger population and they are much more likely to experience poverty."[7]

I might have been the only disabled woman who bought a home through Patti, our realtor. Even then, I only closed the deal; I didn't pay for it.

I took ownership of the unit next door. I may not have paid for it, but I felt the moral responsibility to take care of it. I got the mail and let Maria know if there was anything important for her. She had notified the appropriate agencies about her move, but something always gets by. I emailed her about a package that came from an environmental group; it was obviously soliciting donations, but I wanted to check if there was anything worth keeping before I discarded it. I made a resolution at New Years that I would not buy any greeting cards. I figure I have enough cards in my card box; all I need to do is cross out the inappropriate message and write a new one in. I know it is not the most aesthetically pleasing thing to do, but since we are living on a dying planet, I figure recycling cards is the least I can do. I don't have any grandiose notion that it will solve the problem, but we all need to change our expectations. This is my little public service announcement: We don't need to bother joining consumer culture and buying a product that will probably just be recycled. We can instead make better choices if we use what we already have. In Maria's mail there was a stack of cards from the environmental group. I picked out an appropriate card for my niece Maddy's 15th birthday; it was a polar bear. If I had not used it, it would have only taken up space at the landfill.

I also got the mail that came for my father to that unit. He got the notice of condo fees. I would email him about any mail that arrived for him, and he could direct me on whether I should open it or simply forward it on to his Vegreville address. If I knew it was important, I simply opened the mail and emailed him copies of the contents. I know opening someone's mail is a federal offence, but I thought he would be lenient. A website developed by the Toronto Defence Lawyers states, "Before wireless correspondence, everything came in the mail. Because of this, the Canada Post Corporation Act makes it illegal for any unauthorized individual to open, keep or even delay someone else's mail."[8] If Dad wanted to take me to court, I would depend on him to pay the lawyers' fees, so it seemed that it would have been a ridiculous effort. I figured opening the condo fees letter wasn't too personal.

Getting Permission from the Condo Board

I received an email from Carrie of ILNS that said:

> I sent a correspondence to all participants today, giving an update on where we are at in the pilot.
>
> I'm updating you and Vicky a bit differently as we have a different relationship and I feel I can be completely transparent. We are getting push back from the condo board. First, they asked for a building engineer to review the plans and cited a particular by-law. They also wanted assurances that the changes wouldn't decrease the value of the surrounding units. As you may recall, we reached out to [the contact with the condo corporation] in September to tell her our intentions and to request floor plans. When we followed up on Tuesday, we told them that we had reconnected with Habermehl [our contractor] and the architect and construction team had verified that there were no changes to structure with either unit, verified that HRM (Halifax Regional Municipality) did not require a building engineer to sign off on the changes and that we hoped they would reconsider.

To that end, they replied today to inform us that the request has gone to the corporation's solicitor and building engineer and from there they will make a final decision. Additionally, they feel that ILNS should make a presentation to the board to explain the intended "use" of these units. It has been clearly explained to them that these units will have four individuals who live with severe physical disabilities, living in them and sharing attendant care. I also explained that it was the intention of ILNS to purchase these units at the end of the pilot and the individuals would remain living there, in community as they should. They understand the intent and I am completely mystified as to why they want to go down this rabbit hole. I've been in contact with Claire McNeil [a lawyer with the Disability Rights Coalition] who is willing to represent our interest in this matter. She's reviewing everything and has suggested that it may be a good idea if we can find out who sits on the board. Do you have a listing of who is on the board and how to contact them? We are all in agreement that we need to do an in-person presentation to them as soon as possible. When talking with Habermehl today, they expect permits in the next 10 days. I have been working on this shitshow since first thing this morning. I've also talked to Vicky. Her comments involved something about ableist asses ... lol.

I sent Carrie the email addresses of the board members I knew. We had the Charter of Rights and Freedoms on our side. They could take it to their lawyers, but we are not doing anything beyond what we are legally permitted to do. They can say that it is a family building, but how do you define a family? There was no problem with me living in the unit and having roommates. There is also a unit on the second floor that is rented to four international students. I don't know when the building became family oriented, but it must have changed after I bought my unit. I would think they would have to vote on that. I don't remember any information being circulated about that. I also know that no information was passed along to us when the unit was purchased. (I took law when I was at planning school. I was the top kid in my class.)

HRM is working on changing the land-use by-laws to make group homes possible in any district in HRM; a preliminary report has been written by HRM staff. So, even if we were trying to put in a group home, which we are not, it would be allowable.

At the lawyer's suggestion we sent a new copy of the request for permission to alter from my parents, the actual owners of the two units. The request was approved without delay. No presentation was required. I guess we had nothing to worry about.

I will not swear at the condo board even though that is how I might feel.

Bob the Builder

"I bet you get endless jokes about Bob the Builder," I commented to the head of the renovations.

"You can't even imagine, I've heard them all, probably twice," replied Bob.

The renovations we were making to the two condos were not for aesthetic purposes. They were to make the condos more accessible. We were lowering the counter in the kitchen and getting appliances that were more disability friendly. We were getting a double door fridge so both the freezer and the refrigerator were accessible to someone in a power chair. The stove needed controls at the front of the unit rather than at the back where they are unreachable to someone in a chair. The two bathrooms were reconfigured. Rather than there being two bathtubs, we would have one half bathroom with only a toilet and the washing machine. The other bathroom is being totally tiled so it can be used both as a shower room and as a place to get changed. The doorways to the bedrooms needed to be widened. The doorway into the kitchen needed to be made wider. (I had already widened the kitchen doorway in my unit. There was a flood in my kitchen when one of the pipes in the wall behind the stove burst. We had to replace all the flooring in the kitchen and front entry. Because we were doing that, I thought it was a perfect time to widen the doorway.) There is a single step up to a patio in both the main room and the master bedroom. (I had bought a small ramp that I could use to navigate the step.) The Shared Attendant Program could do better than that. I also was closing off the master bedroom in my unit and putting in a new doorway. I wanted to keep my closet. In exchange I was willing to sacrifice the hallway. By making a new entry way into the bedroom from the main room, we could drive my chair more easily. Right now, there is not enough room for the driver of my chair to fit comfortably between the foot of my bed and the wall. With a new door it will be better.

I wanted to yell at Bob because the job was running behind schedule. But I knew the delays were not his fault; it was the whole industry.[9] William Hrynewich, an estimator with Roof Master, an Ottawa roofing company, said in CBC article from June 2022 that "the labour shortage began early in the pandemic. Add supply shortages and shipping bottlenecks, and the industry has been working at capacity for some time now."[10]

Things in Nova Scotia are no different. If I had a son or daughter, I would encourage them to go into the construction field, and I think the Nova Scotia Community College should take more students. I know Dalhousie is confident it will expand the campus even further; the school recently bought and tore down four houses on Coburg Street, another 15 houses on Robie Street, and one on Edward Street, probably for residences. Where are all the students coming from? And why are they going to university? If they took up a trade, they might actually find employment. There is also a shortage of care workers. No one is looking for someone with a BA in sociology — I speak from experience!

If the whole construction system is messed up, it makes sense why the tiling that Kathleen ordered for the bathroom is out of stock with no date for when it might be available. We will simply have to pick another tile even if it is fourth or fifth in our choices. How important is the colour of our tile anyhow? I don't plan to spend an inordinate amount of time in the bathroom. But maybe if I had a bowel condition or if I planned to shower a lot, I would feel differently. Right now, I am trying to buy a shower chair on Facebook Marketplace. I had used a tray to wash my hair. I didn't have a shower chair because the former bathroom was not accessible and having a bath was hard on the backs of my care workers, although I did have a lift that would allow me to do that. There was a shower chair in Saint John, New Brunswick, that would have been perfect, but it sold to someone else.

The contractors want all possessions removed from the unit so they are not held liable if any possessions disappear. Rather than it being my word against theirs, they asked that there be nothing in the unit. I have to move to the recently renovated unit next door so they can take my unit apart. The social worker in charge of the move said I have to pay $200 for the move. I was impressed by that amount. I am used to scrounging boxes from the local super-markets and liquor stores. I hired a guy the last time I used before in anticipation of the move as I knew I would need someone to move the dresser and couch. Tom used to be my mule but since he fractured his vertebra, he is less reliable. What the social worker failed to tell me was that the cost of taking apart and reassembling my bed was over and above the $200.

I am lucky that one of my assistants loves to pack. While I think of packing as monotonous and repetitive, she loves it. Her fiancé is strong and tall. He has already been "voluntold" he will help. I am glad to give responsibility to someone else. I am amused by how little I am interested in packing. If I need to find anything I am happy enough to text her and have her give me directions on where to find certain items.

I think the people in my building have too much time on their hands. My assistant brought me a letter that had been posted on the door of the unit next to mine, which read, "Awful!" I figure if someone had enough time to write the note and post it on the door, they have enough time to grab a dust buster and clean up the wood shavings in the hallway. If I were an observer, I would think, given all the work that was being done on the unit, that there was likely no one living there. I thought I would clean up the shavings. The dust buster I owned was no longer recharging, so I checked the price of a new one at Canadian Tire and I thought that the price was exorbitant. Instead, I went to Facebook Marketplace. I had two assistants working because one was still training. I asked the assistant in training if he would mind going to pick up a new-to-me vacuum; he was then off to Dartmouth. The woodchips were gone in an instant. I recycled the letter.

The photographs on the next few pages follow a clockwise direction around the condo. All photos are by Nicola Davison, Snickerdoodle Photography.

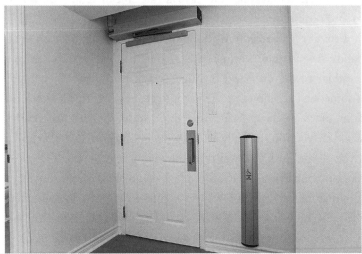

Automatic door opener that can be activated by a power chair user simply by driving into it.

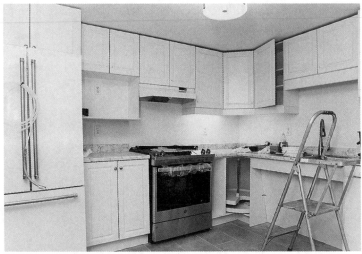

Accessible kitchen appliances.

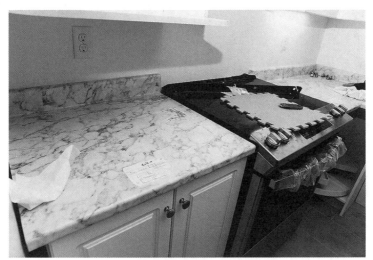

The stove is useable by someone in a wheelchair by having the burner controls in the front rather than at the back.

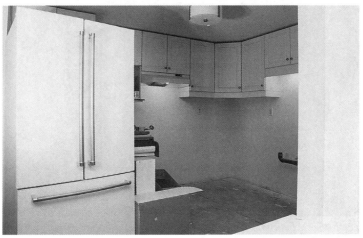

The kitchen as it was being built. The accessible refrigerator has the freezer at the bottom instead of at the top.

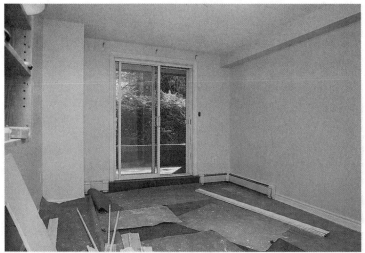

One of the bedrooms still under construction. It was painted in blue, a colour chosen by a participant.

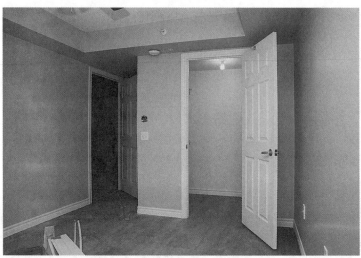

The finished bedroom features enlarged doors for easier access. The closet door maintained its original width.

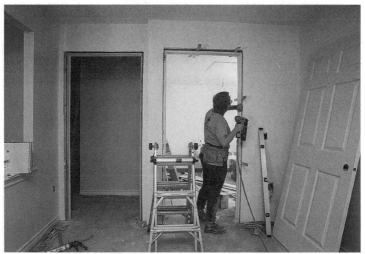

A worker with the contractors touches up the door frame in the bed-room closet.

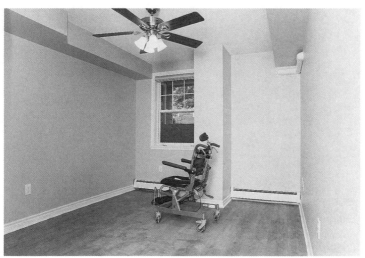

A finished bedroom.

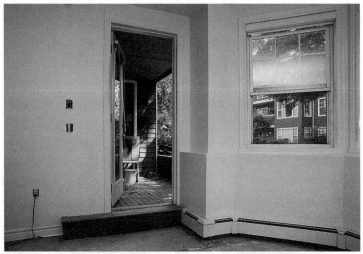

The main room looking out onto the patio and beyond that into the backyard. The step onto the patio was removed and will later be replaced with a lift.

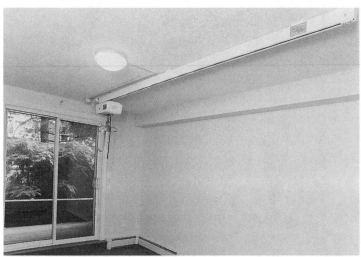

The master bedroom features a patio door to the backyard and a lift.

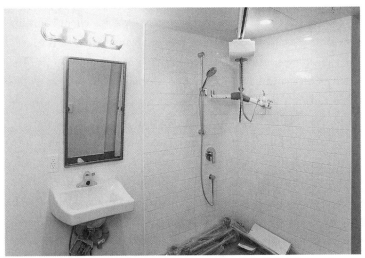

The roll-in shower and lift. Tubs were removed and the shower is accessible with a lift. The sink is operated with an automatic motion sensor which has a water temperature set to warm.

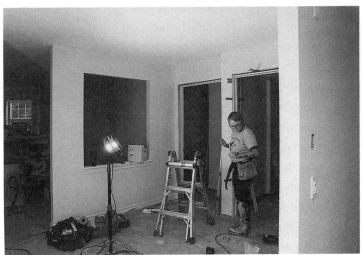

Looking from the main room into the shower room and bedroom, the contractor puts the finishing touches on the paint.

Choosing Participants

The Department of Health and Wellness asked the client coordinators for every client between the ages of 18 and 49 in HRM to see if their clients would be interested in living in the community. That is why Carrie and I had not been comfortable with Edelstein's idea of recruiting candidates for living at his building on Gottingen; there was a waitlist, and we didn't want to interfere with that.

The health files of the 12 interested people were then sent to Carrie and Kathleen at ILNS. From the 12, they had to pick three clients whose care needs would be appropriate with mine.

Joanne Larade, who had muscular dystrophy, was going to be one of the people who lived in the new unit, but unfortunately, she passed away on Tuesday, May 14, 2019.[11] Joanne was 47, too young to be in a nursing home. She had been a great advocate for people with disabilities who were forced to go into nursing homes long before they should have been (if anyone should ever have to go into a nursing home).

I wrote myself into the proposal so that if we were successful in getting a pilot program, I would be included. Maybe that was crass of me, but I think of it as planning ahead. I am a licensed professional planner. Planning is what I do.

I am glad that choosing participants was not up to me. If we were still meeting at Sagewood in Lower Sackville, the four participants in the meetings would have been the obvious choices for the Shared Attendant Program. It would have been me, Vicky Levack, Melanie Gaunt and Joanne Larade. By the time we were ready, Melanie Gaunt also was not an option because she was no longer living in a nursing home. She had decided that she could look after herself with the help of homecare.

Kathleen and Carrie didn't have fun going through the files. It took nearly three weeks. They realized that they had the lives of three people in their hands. The first consideration had to be whether the shared program would meet their individual needs. The second consideration was whether that individual would be compatible with the other participants.

The first participant they chose was Vicky Levack. She had been working on getting out of a nursing home and other disability rights issues for years.[12] Carrie and Kathleen thought the choice was obvious. A quick search of the internet found thirteen articles featuring Vicky on six separate sites. When I was researching, I found her in four journal articles — not about her directly but places that have her voice. Her most recent work is on sexual violence and the institutional control of disabled people's sexuality.[13]

The other two participants were harder to choose. I asked Carrie about non-female candidates. I was told there were a few, but all were deemed to be incompatible for personality reasons.

That means that the other two participants are female. We were supposed to meet via Zoom, but one of the participants had problems with her laptop and ILNS could not enter the long-term care facility to try remedy the situation because of COVID-19 rules. I read the document from the Government of Nova Scotia titled "COVID-19 Management in Long Term Care Facilities. Directive Under the Authority of the Chief Medical Officer of Health." I found a number of ways which I think Kathleen could have used to have the participant leave the building with the offensive laptop. But I might be taking a loose definition of "appointment" and "visitor"; maybe the person who was selected for the Shared Attendant Program has a tighter understanding of the words than I do. Then I heard a CBC Radio broadcast on *Information Morning* on June 23, 2022, about how the administrators of nursing homes aren't actually following the guidelines of the chief medical officer. The woman being interviewed had both of her parents pass away recently in long-term care. She had not been able to visit her father in person until he had lost the mental capacity to recognize her.

Maybe getting in to fix the participant's laptop really was impossible. Maybe we really couldn't meet online.

Living on Our Own

Some of the participants in the program may have gone directly from living with their parents to a nursing home. I wondered how their parents felt about them moving into the community. I thought they would be both excited and terrified. I know that I am.

You know that at a nursing home, the amount of trouble your little angel can get involved in is limited. For a start, all the meals are prepared. You do not need to worry that she will eat only potato chips and cookies for her meals. I eat via feeding tube. I am able to chew and swallow with an increasing amount of difficulty. I am okay with ice cream and pudding. I used to be okay with the middle of perogies and the inside of vine leaves. I am not allowed to have oatmeal, nuts or coconut because they do not break down with saliva. I can have oat milk and coconut flavour, just not the pieces. I was angry when I lost the ability to eat the foods that I liked to prepare. Cooking was a staple activity of my date nights with Tom. I thought things would be ruined if I could no longer dine with Tom. But Tom said that things would change as they had to.

I was lucky that my mother taught me early on how to prepare in advance to achieve proper nutrition. But as I grew up in a rural area, things may have been a bit different. I am a vegetarian now, but my family would buy half a steer and thirty chickens directly from the farmers that produce them. We would have enough vegetables frozen from the gardening season to last most of the year. We had two large freezers in the basement.

I have lived on my own since moving into residence at university. I lived in two different dormitories. In neither did I have to share a room. I liked eating at the cafeteria. They always had food prepared. I know that the food in nursing homes may not be spectacular, but at least it is already prepared.

Parents have enough on their mind trying to deal with the empty nest syndrome. However, their children may not have learned how to buy their own groceries or make a meal plan for a week or a month in advance. They will have to learn that as part of the Shared Attendant Program. Unlike at nursing homes, there is no dietician on staff.

However, the nursing home is not risk free; it presents its own cauldron of trouble. According to the 2019 stats from Statistics Canada, the violence in nursing homes is overwhelming. Although the figures available were for the senior population, the numbers for non-seniors would be similar if not higher. If the rate for sexual assault amongst over 65-year-old women was 20%, I can only imagine that it is higher for the younger women who are particularly vulnerable.

First Impressions

On Saturday, December 4, 2021, I found out the play I was attending ended at 9:35 p.m. I had booked my Access-A-Bus for 9:30 p.m. I was worried Access-A-Bus might go without me if I didn't leave the theatre at the intermission and wait for the bus. I have been on Access-A-Bus before when a client was left for not being ready on time. But the show Tom and I went to was being put on by Zuppa Theatre, a company I had done two plays with (they were nonspeaking roles).

One of the ticket takers at the show was a woman who had worked at one of the shows I was in. She offered to call Access-A-Bus for me and tell them I would be five minutes late. The other person on the bus was Vicky Levack; she had been at the Convention Centre reciting a poem she wrote. Tom asked the driver if I could sit on the bus facing backwards so I could chat with Vicky. She answered him in the negative. I had to sit facing forward.

We drove to my building. Vicky announced to the driver, a woman with long blonde hair named Shayla, that she would soon be living in the building same as me. I didn't ever think about how I would react to this kind of news. I was proud. I thought it was amazing that Vicky had such good news to share.

Vicky thought that the building looked "swanky." First impressions leave a lasting mark. I remember the first time I met Tom. He was helping a friend of his with a video screening of non-verbal animated films for the refugee sponsorship group that I was a part of. The person leading the project had brought Tom in for technical assistance.

I remember my first impression of the condo building 13 years ago. It has two large planters outside the front door. I thought they should be replaced with a bike rack, which would encourage residents to be more sustainable. A visual reminder is always a good thing. Remember, I used to be the transportation coordinator at an environmental organization. Just because I can't use a bicycle doesn't mean I shouldn't encourage it in other people!

Tom's boss thought that the building I lived in was some sort of seniors assisted living residence. I don't know if that is a good thing or bad. I wonder why he and his wife thought that... I am sure it is those damn planters that give that idea. They look like something my grandmother would appreciate. When Vicky visited my unit, she thought that it was spacious and that the building is nice with wide hallways. She is more polite than to comment on my decorating capacity or lack thereof. She was worried about running over the cats with her wheelchair. I said, "They will learn soon enough to stay out of your way."

Interdependence and Autonomy

Like most other teenagers, the greatest goal I had was to finally become independent. I didn't want to rely on my parents anymore. I wanted to be my own person. Little did I realize that my goal should not have been independence, but autonomy. The more I think about it, even if I am dependent on people financially and physically, I can still be an independent thinker.

Most people are interdependent, not independent, unless of course, you make your own bread and harvest your own fruits and vegetables from your own greenhouse. More people than ever are going off-grid, so I do not doubt that is possible for you to be one of those people. Making your own materials for the greenhouse is a little trickier, but I will not question you.

Many people are dependent on bakers for their morning loaves. I don't have toast for breakfast, but I do depend on the producers of my Promote tube feed and the truckers who bring the food from the warehouse in Ontario, and if we go further back, I am dependent on the government that pays for the roads and the people who laid it and the company that produced the paint to make the dotted white lines and the shoulders, and the car manufacturer and the steel plant. As a society we are quite interwoven.

When we are young adults why don't we learn about interdependence not independence? I don't really understand why the goal of our society is not about interdependence. I know I am much happier depending on my partner to make me laugh, rather than how I would feel if I depended on a comedian on Netflix. I also don't know how the comedian would help me solve my problems; I have written to celebrities before, and usually they don't reply. Tom knows better than to simply ignore me. At least I hope he does.

In the article "Relational Autonomy in Assisted Living: A Focus on Diverse Care Settings for Older Adults," the authors Molly Perkin, Mary Ball and Frank Whittington say, "A relational self is both individuated and interdependent and viewed as emerging out of relationships with other individuals, social groups, and institutions, which may either support or oppress one's opportunities for self-direction, self-discovery, and self-definition."[14] The individual is a person in and of themselves, but they require a larger social situation for them to realize their being. In the Shared Attendant Program, I hope there is enough diversity of staff and other participants to ensure this happens. However, there is room for everyone to have time in the community with support if the program does not offer enough to the participants.

According to Perkin et al., "maintaining an authentic self will not be easy." They write, "Across studies, analysis shows that maintaining an authentic sense of self in the everyday world of AL [assisted living] is a constant struggle. Loss is a recurring theme in residents' accounts of their transition into AL and their ensuing lives." But because losses should not be a common occurrence of the Shared Attendant Program (I hope), participants will feel more like their authentic selves.

An autonomous individual can rely on others both to have their care needs fulfilled and to maintain their independence. An individual in Nova Scotia may not get a large choice in long-term care facilities, but they do get to choose between facilities. Now that the Shared Attendant Program is in operation, the choice is larger if they are between the ages of 18 and 49. It is important to maintain social connections within the community. Having participants live within the community is critical to them remaining autonomous.

Vulnerable

"So, it wasn't a matter of *if* I would be raped, it was a matter of when," says Vicky Levack in an interview with one of my assistants on April 27, 2022, referring to the recent attack she experienced. The rate of sexual assault on women with disabilities in

Canada is twice the rate of that for able-bodied women, which is about 30% according to Statistics Canada.[15] For disabled women in Nova Scotia, a government report entitled *Sexual Violence: A Public Health Primer* puts the number closer to 2.5 times higher.[16] In other words, nearly 75% of women with disabilities in Nova Scotia are sexually assaulted, not just 60%.

I put a rod in my screen door to stop it from being opened more than a couple of inches; I figure that no man (expect Inspector Gadget using his Go-Go Gadget arms) could get the rod out (and Inspector Gadget is a good guy so he wouldn't do such a thing). I live on the main floor of the condo building. Since the start of COVID-19, Tom has been living with me, but my voice is so little that only if the baby monitor is on and is close to me is there any way that he could hear me. It doesn't matter how loud I try to yell; it barely registers as a sound. I am a sitting duck. I know Tom would fight to the death for me, but he would be 30 feet away and oblivious if anything were to happen.

Feminists have said the stranger-rapist is so uncommon that it's almost a myth, though I can't help but be scared of Paul Bernardo types. It's much more common to be assaulted by someone you know. So with the rod, I guess I only need to worry about that. It is not the total solution, but it is a piece.

If that is not scary enough, according to the US Department of Justice Office for Victims of Crime, 20% of crime victims with disabilities in the US believed they were targeted because of their disability.[17] Individuals with disabilities are particularly vulnerable to crime for a variety of reasons, including but not limited to reliance on caregivers, limited transportation options, limited access to sign language interpreters and assistive devices, and isolation from the community.

For Vicky, her experience had a profound effect. In our interview, she said, "That girl who really enjoyed her sexuality and reveled in it, died that day. And [was] replaced by a woman who is very hurt. And, very scared. I am trying to get [the woman who reveled in her sexuality] back, but it's going to take some time. I think it's going to be something I'll be working on my entire life actually to get back to, if I'm being honest."

It is interesting that one of the first comments Carrie made to me about the new unit was that the doors would be locked at all times. I think that is a wise move. Since Vicky's rape, she is understandably not interested in fooling around. That leaves the other members of the adjacent units in a pickle. Part of me wants to reject all notion of love in solidarity with Vicky, but I don't think she would want that. I think she would want me to be more like the person she was before the assault.

Assisted Sex

ILNS decided not to go with my suggestion of putting assisted sex in the contract for caregivers. Assisted sex is not surrogacy. It is being willing to help clients get into lingerie for an upcoming participant date or getting a participant into positions for sex with their partner(s) or self or helping a quadriplegic insert a vibrator.[18] But ILNS wisely thought that given Nova Scotia's shortage of care workers, it was better not to put anything in the contract that was out of the ordinary.

I see why ILNS left it up to the individual care worker to decide if they were okay with participating. Attendants have sexual rights, which include the right to a workplace that is not sexualized. Assisted sex gets tricky when (monogamous) partners and the like are involved. If participants in the Shared Attendant Program want the assistant to engage in such tasks, they could bring it up directly with the worker. ILNS will not discourage the participants from having sex, whether it be with a long-term partner or a casual hookup. Rules for these encounters would need to be carefully laid out, and all parties would need to be okay with the activities.

Research has demonstrated that "sexuality is so very clearly a quality-of-life issue," say Steven Welch and Gerrit Clements in their paper called "Development of a Policy on Sexuality for Hospitalized Chronic Psychiatric Patients."[19] I thought, maybe naively, that helping a quadriplegic set up a vibrator was no more sexual than putting a tampon in. But, speaking to some of my assistants I discovered that people have very different understandings of the subject. I find it interesting how many opinions and how varied they are on subject of putting a vibrator into a participant. Maybe I looked at it from the perspective of a disabled person who is unable to masturbate independently. Maybe I need to think of it like an able-bodied person does. Maybe I should have looked at it as group masturbation.

The Shared Attendant Program was not going to make any outlandish statement while still in the trial period; that was something that could be done when the program was more secure. If you look at how much homecare has changed in the last 50 years, it is not surprising that assisted sex is now an issue. When Kathleen's parents met 34 years ago, male and female clients were divided into separate sections of the care facility. A male attendant could only work with male clients, and thus there was no mixing of genders. I do not think a third or fourth category of sexual/gender orientation existed in common parlance. They did exist, of course, but were not discussed in polite conversation.

When we were setting up the units in the community, my greatest hope was that Tom and I could still sleep together. I think I am the only person in the Shared Attendant Program who has a partner, which means that assisted sexual encounters might be something that the other participants in the program want to explore. I don't know if any of the other participants have the gall and forwardness to raise the issue. I don't think Vicky is in the space to do it. That means I should.

A research study by Cory Silverberg and Fran Odette entitled the Sexuality and Access Project collected individual experiences with attendant services and sexual support. It began with some basic truths that are simple but are often simply ignored: sexual rights are human rights. Sexual health is a core component of general health. People with disabilities who use attendant services have a right to information and resources about their sexual health and support in expressing their sexuality.

There are certain products that the homecare provider may want to purchase and provide to their patrons in order to address the complete needs of their clientele. Or maybe there should be a government grant for products such as Ripple, which is a three-part masturbation suit that is created to satisfy the needs of people with moderate to severe functional limitations. I do not know if the suit works, and I am not endorsing it; I'm just trying to tell the public that there are solutions out there. We only need to be willing to ask the questions. Asking the questions may seem awkward, but that is only because we don't usually have the conversation.

I asked a friend of mine who works in homecare about sexual support. She was intrigued by the subject. She has not gotten any information from her employer about how to approach the subject of sexual support. Most of her clients are elderly and not interested in intercourse (or so she thinks). The *New York Times*, quoting from a survey of sex and seniors in the United States, says, "Sex and interest in it do fall off when people are in their 70s, but more than a quarter of those up to age 85 reported having sex in the previous year. And the drop-off has a lot to do with health or lack of a partner, especially for women."[20] The study was published in the *New England Journal of Medicine* in 2007.

People seem to assume that sex is something that only young and able-bodied people engage in.[21] Maybe it has to do with women interested in procreating, but in reality things are not quite that simple.

Partner Surrogacy

I have not participated in hook-up culture. Maybe it is due to my Christian upbringing or maybe it is because I grew up in a time when HIV was a death sentence. Or maybe it is because I have only slept with men I love. Regardless, I think that the connection I have with sexual partners is a real thing and that it can be during hook-ups as well.

I don't know how sexual surrogacy works on an emotional level. According to Wikipedia, "Sex surrogates, sometimes referred to as surrogate partners, are practitioners trained in addressing issues of intimacy and sexuality. A surrogate partner works in collaboration with a sex therapist to meet the goals of their client. This triadic model is used to dually support the client: the client engages in experiential exercises and builds a relationship with their surrogate partner while processing and integrating their experiences with their therapist and clinician."

I mean, I can see how theoretically it is easy for one to separate the physical act of sex from the emotional component. Maybe I just have not slept around enough. I don't know what a sex worker feels for their clients. I am sure that a sexual partner surrogate could have the same division. A sexual surrogate has both asexual and relational interactions with their clients.

In the two films I watched about surrogacy, *Private Practices: The Story of a Sexual Surrogate* and *The Sessions*,[22] the worker did have some emotional connection with the clients. But it was Hollywood. I want to talk with an actual surrogate before I draw any conclusions. The emails I sent to surrogates were unanswered.

There is only one sexual surrogate in Halifax, where I reside, that I could find; there might be more that don't advertise and are not known to the groups I contacted. I also emailed some people in California.

In calling around about sexual partner surrogacy, I learned to be careful with the word surrogacy and preface my statements with, "I am a quadriplegic and I need help to masturbate." That way, I didn't automatically get referred to a fertility clinic. I have heard the term "medically assisted sex" used to describe persons with severe physical disabilities getting help in securing sex. That phrase reminds the world that sex is a part of treating the whole person. Sex might be a taboo subject, but it is as natural as defecating. Why do we treat it differently?

Being a Good Roommate

My soon-to-be roommate asked me about furniture and if I wanted anything new. She had already bought new small appliances for the kitchen and asked if I minded. I told her that the kitchen was Tom's domain, and I didn't think he would have a problem with new toys. "I don't spend any time in the kitchen, and if you want new gadgets, then go for it." When she asked about living room furniture, it was a different story.

I bought a futon second-hand before the bedbug crisis hit Halifax. At that time no one had ever heard of a bedbug much less be hesitant to buy used furniture because of their existence. I now insist that any furniture with fabric be new. I was a member of a couple of refugee settlement organizations who had to change the way they operated because of bedbugs. No longer could we rely on second-hand furniture so we could focus the limited dollars we raise on other settlement costs, such as rent. I had already given Vicky the lecture on "only new items that have fabric." She was receptive to my ideal. When she asked about buying a couch, my immediate response was no. I had survived with a loveseat and a futon for thirteen years. The planet is dying. I certainly do not need to add yet another piece of trash to the landfill. I worked for the Ecology Action Centre for too long not to be indoctrinated into thinking about sustainability.

Then I thought about it more. Tom had fractured a vertebra and was using the futon as a bed in the room that would soon be Vicky's. The futon had a broken leg and was being propped up by a stack of literature. I didn't think it was suitable for the living room. I didn't think the loveseat was big enough for Tom. He is about 72 inches long. He was 6 feet 2 inches but with the compression of his spine as he ages and his tendency to slouch, I figure it is less now. However, with the loveseat being only 45 inches, it is clearly not big enough.

Maybe I was thinking about it in the wrong way. Vicky had been in a nursing home for a decade, and a nicer, more considerate roommate might simply agree to the couch because it was Vicky's first real home. I wasn't willing to cater to her disabled status that way. Maybe I should be kinder but the planet… Maybe I am just unfamiliar with being a roommate. I used to have a sign on my bedroom door that read "The Boss." I was used to having ten to fourteen employees to do my bidding. I was used to setting the rules.

I thought the "shy cherry" colour we had used to paint the front entry might be a little dated, so I looked on the Benjamin Moore website for something more current. "Wild flower" was lovely, and it would paint well over the colour that was there. I didn't even think to consult Vicky even though it was now also her apartment. I will need to change my ways. I have been living alone for some time. Even after Tom moved in, he lets me think I am the boss. It will be a steep curve to learn humility.

Department of Seniors and Long-Term Care

Nothing happens in government without a reason. Nova Scotia's population is aging. The average age is 44.2 according to Statistics Canada. The 2021 census shows that 22.2% of the total population is 65 and older — shocking.[23]

I find it amusing that the Shared Attendant Program is under the Department of Seniors and Long-Term Care because we are neither seniors nor are we in long term care. We are between the ages of 18 and 49, and we live in the community. In fact, the recommendations of an expert advisory panel on long-term care explicitly states young people should have specific programming because "their physical, psychological, and educational needs differ from the majority of older residents."[24]

That is not to say that seniors in long-term care don't deserve our attention. After COVID-19 became a pandemic, the problems in nursing homes were highlighted. Because the virus had not been seen before, people in nursing homes had no immunity to it and were hit particularly hard. The death rate from COVID-19 in nursing homes in Canada was 81%, the highest in the world, says the Science Application Forum in an article called "Restoring Trust: COVID-19 and the Future of Long-Term Care in Canada."[25]

This has led to some advocating for long-term care to be nationalized, as most homes are currently run by private corporations for profit. "Nationalizing long-term care, sometimes referred to as publicizing the system, would undoubtedly take profits out of long-term care and may create system-wide changes to improve residents' conditions," say authors Kelley Fritsch and Fady Shanouda in an article arguing to nationalize homecare instead of long-term care.[26] Nursing homes are often looked at with scorn. They are not places where people want to live. However, they are places where some people have to live. They are seen as a last resort. But this ignores the reasons why they are hated.

The argument to nationalize long-term care disregards the "fundamental character of long-term care facilities as an extension of the carceral state, essentially prisons by a different name," Fritsch and Shanouda say. The same article refers to the fact that residents of long-term care are not able to decide when or if they will shower or bathe, when or what they will eat and when they will go to bed or get up in the morning. If you are in long term care, you will likely be separated from your partner or spouse. You will likely only have your dietary needs accommodated if you are persistent about it, and it helps if you have medical documentation; if not, you eat what you get.

We must ask if publicizing a broken system is worth it, or if fundamental changes need to happen. Institutionalized systems do not give individuals the freedom of choice. They are not appropriate for younger or middle-aged adults with severe disabilities. Clients are shut in the facility; this has only gotten worse with COVID-19. According to the article mentioned above, they are often administered psychotropic medication (chemical restraints), locked in their rooms and placed in physical restraints. The workers in long-term care facilities earn a meagre amount. Their work is physically demanding, they are required to work precarious hours, and they are always risking injury or illness. They may need to work at more than one facility to earn enough to live on.

Fritsch and Shanouda discuss two recent high-profile examples of younger adults with physical disabilities that made the news — one in Manitoba, the other in Quebec. These individuals felt like they gave up their lives to the system. The individual in Quebec "camped out in a makeshift cage on the lawn of Québec's National Assembly in August 2020." The person in Manitoba built a mock jail cell in downtown Winnipeg "to protest the way in which the Manitoba care system locked him out of his own life."[27] They both wanted to draw attention to how North America needs to review how it deals with seniors and people with complex care needs. The way things are currently done leaves a segment of society without the care it deserves. Maybe that is not the best long-term strategy. Maybe the current system needs change.

I thought that, at least for seniors, multi-generational living situations could help. That way the entire family could help; in multi-generational apartments (versus single-family units as is the norm in Canada), there could be more people of various ages around to cook and clean. But it does not recognize the realities in a country as large and individualized as Canada. I don't know how 24/7 care would work. Instead, the Shared Attendant Program has a lot of possibilities.

It is doubtful that we will be able to eliminate long-term care facilities all together. I know that with my grandmother, although my mother lived down the street from her, there was a point where it wasn't safe for her to be living on her own. She went to an assisted living facility. When she got really ill, she had to go into hospital. All three of her children cared about her welfare, but only one of them was willing to spend time long term with her. One was living in another province, one in a different community. Neither wanted to run the family farm. My mother's husband was happy to take on the task. But neither myself nor my sister wanted to enter the farming lifestyle. I had been quite enamoured by the country life as a child but ended up moving across the country for school and I live in a condo in the heart of Halifax. My sister who had never given the farm a second look now lives on an acreage and maintains a handful of chickens.

There will always have to be a place for people with complex care needs who have no other option. But that doesn't mean we should not repurpose some homes if we can figure out how to get more people living in the community with the supports they need.

Continuing Care Assistants

On the January 11, 2022, the Halifax *CityNews* reported, "Katelyn Randell, director of long-term care, told the [Nova Scotia] legislature's health committee Tuesday that 25 of the 133 nursing homes are not accepting new admissions as they address what she called 'staffing gaps.'"[28] How was the Shared Attendant Program ever going to attract the needed continuing care assistants (CCAs) if established nursing homes could not get all the staff they needed?

The major problem is the rate of pay. The job of continuing care assistants is physically demanding and has impossible hours. Employees often get injured.[29] In order to acquire this position, they have to be certified by the province. On top of that, they earn a pittance. According to *novascotia.ca*, the annual salary for a CCA increased to a final amount of between $44,660 and $48,419 in February 2022.[30] You require a college education to be a CCA. Anne-Marie Slaughter, author of the book *Unfinished Business*, says, "What's really going on here is we are discriminating against people who have to care for others, which is a role that society needs people to play."[31]

When I read in an email from Carrie that the Shared Attendant Program is not using continuing care assistants, I could hear the refrain of "Somewhere Over the Rainbow" echo through my head. I had spent countless nights wondering how we were going to attract CCAs from the already limited pool in Nova Scotia. Also, according to the *Halifax Examiner* in "Nursing Home Workers Are Moving between Multiple Facilities. That's a Big Problem," CCAs had been accused of spreading COVID-19 between institutions.[32] I didn't want them bringing it here. I shouldn't have been worried. ILNS never planned to use CCAs. Because ILNS was the service provider of the Shared Attendant Program, it was responsible for staff and scheduling.

Carrie wrote in her email in June 22, 2022, that we would be hiring residential resource workers (RRWs). It was a term that was unfamiliar to me, but I guess it is common in the right circles. I guess there needs to be more than one kind of caregiver. Not everyone can earn a college degree and nor can everyone afford it. There is no program for RRWs at the Nova Scotia Community College, but maybe there ought to be. Kathleen explained in her email of June 30, 2022, "In my experience, and likely in your own as someone who has hired attendants, more training doesn't always provide the best fit. It has often been my experience that hiring for soft skills and a willingness to learn and follow directions has been more fruitful than looking for a completed course."

RRWs are legitimately needed, but this does not guarantee they are recognized. They are commonly used by group homes and do not command the same sort of salary as continuing care assistants. RRWs typically get from $18 to $20.68 per hour, but the salaries for both the RRWs and CCAs are too low. As most people doing this kind of care work are women, the low pay is also a gender issue.

Carrie and Kathleen from ILNS reached out to me for recommendations on the people I used for my assistants. I hire a lot of students, but there are other people who are interested in working for the program longer-term. The people I get are open books. Although they have no previous experience in dealing with people with disabilities, they are happy to learn. Because I am the only employer they have had for this kind of thing, my way is the only way they know. They are willing to get trained in the core competencies. The core competencies required to be an RRW can be acquired through individual courses in the community. They involve basic First Aid and cardiopulmonary resuscitation (CPR), fire and life safety awareness, including hazard recognition, being cognizant of medication and its effects, crisis intervention, being alert about triggers, dignity and respect of client information, and mindfulness of proper body mechanics, behavioural supports and individual program planning. Much of the information is client and organization specific.

The program was set to open in about a month. Deadlines were coming hard and fast. Hiring must happen soon. Vicky and I wanted to have some input on hiring. Vicky has spent over a decade in a nursing home not being consulted on who is doing her care. She was stuck in a medicalized system. She was consistently being told what would be done. She was never asked. It was important for her to be consulted now.

I suggested that Carrie ask the four participants for the qualities they thought were the most important for their care, and I wanted to have a mechanism for participants to complain about people who were already hired. I had been in charge of my own hiring for the last decade. I chose all the questions I would ask and decided if I wanted to hire each person. I know the Shared Attendant Program is not Self-Managed Care, but I think participants should still have some input into who is hired.

We worked out a system where the four participants in the program would give ILNS feedback on what was important to them. In a June 23, 2022, email to all participants, we read:

> While ILNS is the service provider, you are the experts in your care. We will refer to you to ensure we know what we should look for in new ILNS employees. Everyone must remember that this is not Self-Managed Care. It is the Shared Services Program, in which, as a service provider, we will facilitate the staffing and scheduling of staff. There is an official complaint process, so you, as the care recipients, will have an avenue to bring forward concerns of any nature promptly. This information will become very clear as each person transitions to the community.

And Kathleen mentioned the following in her email of June 30, 2022:

> As a service provider ILNS has obligations both to the participants and to the attendants as employees. ILNS process will include training, a probationary period, reviews, and a progressive discipline process aligned with best human resource practices. I am confident that once we get the right attendants in place (ones who want to engage in IL [independent living] and understand the importance of self-direction) and retain them, the relationships will be built. I recognize that attendant supports are a delicate balance in that the relationship must remain professional but often personal relationships develop too. On the independent living philosophy and hiring of attendants, when we look at the IL philosophy, it is having things done as we would like them to be done in a way that is respectful of autonomy, choice, and dignity of risk. Carrie, on behalf of ILNS, has ensured IL was included at each step of the way.

I thought that was a positive start. We can make changes as we go. I told ILNS that I thought the most important characteristics for assistants were patience and attention to detail. Patience is needed to use the eye system for my speaking and attention to detail is needed to make sure I do not get a pressure sore. The two questions I wanted ILNS to ask during interviews were:

1. How do you react if you make a mistake?
2. I use a letter system when communicating. I often screw up. How will you react if you have spent a lot of time and effort doing something that turns out to be pointless?

If Vicky and I can contribute to the hiring process, shouldn't we? It might not be possible to have everyone play a role in hiring this time around because of COVID-19, but shouldn't we be setting the framework for that sort of participation? The Shared Attendant Program is a new way of doing things. It is not the medical model.

Disability Support Program

My first meeting with Leah Darton was at the Gottingen Street provincial building, a block away from where the proposed unit with Edelstein would have been built. At the time we did not know whether the plan we had proposed to the Department of Community Services would be approved. I had brought my former boss Mark Butler to the first meeting with a government representative. As he was an experienced government negotiator, I thought he could provide any extra elbow grease we needed. I thought I could use all the help I could get.

Little did I know that Leah was on our side. She was a program coordinator with the Disability Support Program (DSP) at the Department of Community Services. I felt like a church mouse begging at the altar of the provincial government and she was a high priest. But that is not how she saw it.

In her eyes, I was "a city planner, and would know a lot about accessible housing ... an author, an advocate for others ... going to make things happen. I felt like I was going to be on a journey with you and others to see this through. I felt committed to doing my part, to support the Shared Attendant Program to happen."

I interviewed Leah in June 2022. Here are her answers; they have been modified for length and format but not for content.

Jen: *Why do you think Nova Scotia does not have group homes for adults with serious physical impairments?*

Leah: There are Nova Scotians with significant physical impairments living and receiving supports in some DSP homes. Historically, some of the homes that were owned or rented by service providers were nice homes, but older homes with limited accessibility. Some have been modified to become more accessible to support specific participants who were living there who had changing needs, or who were moving in and needed accessibility changes to the home. The commitment to accessibility in Nova Scotia is changing that situation for all Nova Scotians. All new DSP home builds are fully accessible.

In other situations, medical or nursing supports may have been the reason the individual was not supported by the Disability Support Program. Partnerships between government departments, like in the pilot, can provide the opportunity for nursing supports to be in place for participants living in a community setting. The DSP will continue to address these gaps in services for eligible Nova Scotians with physical impairments, with the funding provided to support individuals moving from long-term care to community with the funding provided to expand upon the pilot, and with the funding provided to move individuals out of Disability Support Program facilities.

Jen: *What do you think about the new direction of housing that I proposed?*

Leah: I think your proposal was an exceptional idea which will have far reaching impact. I was so pleased the proposal was accepted and I was able to be a part of the work to see the pilot implemented and the new additional investment for expansion.

Jen: *Why do you think the new model might be more helpful for adults with disabilities?*

Leah: The new shared services model will help to support adults with disabilities to live the lives they choose in their communities. Individual support needs can be met with partnerships in government for shared delivery of services. This will fill a gap in services for individuals with disabilities. I think it will lead the way for programs to be developed in the future and may also inspire other models to be created for shared delivery of services.

Jen: *Do you have any insights into why the waitlists in Nova Scotia for adults with disabilities who need 24-hour care are so long?*

Leah: There was a time when there was little development of small option homes. Currently and over recent years many small option homes have been opened and are continuing to be opened to address the need. Unfortunately, there is some catch-up happening to build and open as fast as possible to meet the need both on the waitlist (service request list) and for those in facilities operated by the Disability Support Program, adult residential centres (ARCs) and regional rehabilitation centres (RRCs) who will also have opportunities to move to smaller settings in community.

Another reason is because Nova Scotia has several ARCs and RRCs over the province, where many individuals needing 24/7 support historically resided. And, as we know, there was an over-reliance on large facilities in Nova Scotia. The service request list (waitlist) is made up of individuals who are currently in other DSP-supported options who want a different option, and those who are waiting for the DSP. There has been recent significant investment in the DSP, which will help to create capacity and lower the amount of individuals waiting for services.

Jen: *How would you like to live in a nursing home? What do you imagine it would be like for you?*

Leah: I would not like to live in a nursing home. I can't imagine that having to be my reality. It's a very medical model and it's not acceptable for young people to live in nursing homes.

Jen: *What do you think needs to be improved with the Department of Community Services?*

Leah: I think DCS needs to modernize the supports and services offered by the Disability Support Program. I believe we are doing that work now, and that advocates (both self-advocates and allies), the sector (those who provide our services), the Department of Community Services, the municipalities and other government departments are moving together in that direction collectively. I believe that will create change, but we have to keep moving forward. More work needs to be done. There has been recent significant investment in the Disability Support Program. This funding will help increase the types of supports we offer and also increase capacity for services. The pilot that was a result of your proposal, as an example, will help to inform future programming in the DSP. There are several initiatives happening that will support reducing the waitlist for services significantly and fill the gaps for some who have not had their support needs met. Once implemented, these changes will improve the Department's supports to individuals with disabilities.

Jen: *How did you become involved in government? Do you have a personal interest in younger adults in nursing homes?*

Leah: I worked for the previous Ministry of Seniors and Community Supports in Alberta. And I worked with individuals in community home settings before that. I began working to support individuals with disabilities early in my adult life and continued along that path. I have both a professional and personal interest in individuals having choice, dignity of risk and opportunities to live the lives they want to live. So, I do try to build that lens into the work.

I am always surprised to hear that government departments did not always work together. To me the government should always be focused on the entire community it serves. I think of the different departments like being the different appendages of the same organism. I think it is crazy for the right hand not to help the left hand if together they could provide a better service for their community. But that is not how things were done in the Nova Scotia government. It is a tremendous change if the departments are all working together. I feel like it is a *kumbaya* moment.

More Waiting

How fast the Shared Attendant Program has come along is entirely a matter of perspective. For Vicky, who can't wait to leave the nursing home, I am sure the project is crawling at a snail's pace. But for me, who is quite happy going to sleep in Tom's arms, the project is moving fast enough. With Tom moving in during COVID-19, he has also been working from home. I have learned a lot about video editing and sound quality. I never knew you had to render video. Now I know. I don't know how the other participants feel.

When I asked Vicky what she wanted kept from the nursing home days, she replied concisely, "Literally nothing. Replicate nothing." I wish I could be as sure of the new project as Vicky is. I have some concerns. I wonder if I will get enough time with my assistants. I am used to being the only item of importance. Now, there will be four of us. I don't share well. I am worried that I won't get enough time with Tom. I am not good on the phone. My voice isn't loud enough to be heard. How will we communicate?

I know I was the one who initiated the project, but that was three years ago. A lot has happened since then. To use Carrie's analogy, her daughter has completed a university degree in the time since the unit was proposed. COVID-19 happened, which meant Tom moved in to do my morning care. I like having him here. Vicky, who will be my roommate, is okay with Tom staying over. She likes Tom. He used to come with me to the meetings of the Empowered group that met at Sagewood. She has asked that I return the favour when she finds a partner. I will do that. But will I have to negotiate how many nights in a row can Tom spend in our shared space? I am not used to having a roommate and having to work things out. I am used to being the boss. Now I will no longer have that kind of role. And maybe I will not have that kind of respect, either.

Vicky is so unhappy at the nursing home that she would go live in a tent in the winter in a public park rather than go back to the nursing home. Vicky says:

I do get disappointed when I hear there's another delay. I do get very sad because trust me, I want to get out of [the nursing home]. I actually threatened to go live in the park that I work at because I felt so unsafe here. I said I'm safer there. I feel safer. But they said if we could accommodate your needs, you could move to the park right now. But they obviously can't accommodate my needs, so I'm forced to stay here. And so, any delay means like, oh, I have to stay here longer, but I know that change is coming and that makes it bearable.

On the other hand, I am ok with the delays. My mom is coming to help me pack and she has not booked her flight yet. So, nothing is really affected by the delays. I bought a fan on Facebook Marketplace when I heard the delays might run into the summer. In my unit there is an air-conditioner in each of the bedrooms. In the new condo there is only air-conditioning in the main room. I don't know if this will affect how cool the unit is, but I got the fan just in case. Anyhow, I think the fan is better for the electricity grid than the air-conditioning. Until Nova Scotia has a reliable source of green energy, I will try to limit my consumption of power.

I was originally told that my roommates would need to vacate their current housing by October 2021. One of my roommates was a student and did not want to be moving in the middle of a semester, so she left in August. It is now months later, and no one has touched the spare room to begin renovation. I was told I would be moving in May. My move is only a couple of months late, at the time of writing this. The delays are expected. The program is new. There are still kinks to be worked out.

Carrie and Kathleen have worked incredibly hard to get the project off the ground.

I received an e-mail from my former neighbour and the old owner of the unit next door, Maria. She asked how the renovations were going. I didn't want her to feel that the sale of her unit was in vain, but I had to admit that the renovations were running behind schedule. The project was delayed yet again. I feel like we are in a baseball game that is perennially in the bottom of the tenth inning. We are almost there, but not quite.

Documenting the Move

I had worked with Rachel Bower before. In 2020, I had run for municipal council, and she made a video about it. Doing another video for Vicky was not a problem. I was happy to be included. They were making a video to be broadcast on the television show *Our Community* on Accessible Media Incorporated (AMI). The video was going to be about how Vicky was successful in her mission to get out of a nursing home. She would be moving in with me when the renovations were finally completed.

I got a text message from Rachel the morning of the shoot. They had arrived on time and had done the first question-and-answer session with Vicky outside in the natural lighting. Rachel and Vicky, along with the crew, had gone to Uncommon Grounds, a local coffee shop. I was disappointed that they didn't go for ice cream. I called Vicky weak because she satisfied her own caffeine addiction before having fun in the warm weather. I didn't want anything from the coffee shop, but I was grateful to be asked.

Rachel wanted some footage of Vicky and I engaging in small talk, but the only problem is that neither Vicky nor I enjoy small talk. But we played the game for Rachel. We sat together in the living room and pretended we were enjoying ourselves. There are too many important issues to discuss to bother wasting time on inane conversation. She wanted us to talk about the small appliances Vicky had purchased. Was I okay with that? I didn't know what I could say, Tom does all the meal prep. Was he okay with new toys? I needed Tom to act as a megaphone and repeat my thoughts. My vocal ability is not much use.

Rachel had envisioned the closing scene being Vicky settling into her new room. Unfortunately, because of construction delays her room would not be ready until long after Rachel's deadline. Rachael had asked for an extension, but it was denied.

I told Rachel I would come up with a closing scene because it was the least I could do — with the small exception of providing bathrooms free of charge to her and her crew. I did not forget about my responsibility, but I have to thank the weather for making it possible. Rachel had mentioned that she wanted to get a shot of Vicky and I travelling side-by-side on the sidewalk. In the residential part of the city the sidewalks are too narrow to go side-by-side. However, by Dalhousie there is the space to do that. There is also room by the Public Gardens. So, I suggested we go on an excursion, which is entirely possible in this part of the city.

We walked to the Public Gardens. I took a somewhat unconventional route, but I have lived in the neighbourhood for over a decade and I find the conventional routes a little boring. So, I go my own way; but I forgot that Vicky does not have the benefit of a personal assistant to drive. Vicky unfortunately did not like the path. Construction blocked the usual return route, but I learned a new way to go, at least when there is no snow. The winter has its own accessibility challenges, but for now I was happy it was summer.

As we were walking Vicky and Rachel asked why I decided not to enter the Gardens at the corner of Spring Garden and Summer Street. I replied that the ice cream is farther along Spring Garden. Why would I choose a route without a reward? The way we went got Rachel the shots she wanted and ended with a great opportunity for interaction. Tom did not really want to be in the video; he is somewhat camera shy. But he got involved with the wrong woman. Tom was willing to be in the video because I needed him to be.

Notes

1. Ericka Dyck, "Institutionalization," Eugenics Archive, December 5, 2014. https://eugenicsarchive.ca/discover/encyclopedia/5482363 5bf64660000000001.
2. MS Society, "Researchers Identify New Potential Genetic Risk Factor for Relapsing-Remitting MS in Women," n.d. https://mssociety.ca/research-news/article/researchers-identify-new-potential-genetic-risk-factor-for-relapsing-remitting-ms-in-women.
3. Centre for Independent Living in Toronto, "What Is Independent Living?" n.d. cilt.ca/about-us/what-is-il/.
4. Giovanni Silvano, "A Brief History of Western Medicine," *Journal of Traditional Chinese Medical Sciences,* 8 (2021). doi.org/10.1016/j.jtcms.2020.06.002.
5. Douglas James Guthrie, "China," Britannica, n.d. britannica.com/science/history-of-medicine/China.
6. Easter Seals, "Disability in Canada: Facts and Figures," n.d. easterseals.ca/wp-content/uploads/2016/12/Disability-in-Canada-Facts-Figures.pdf.
7. Michelle Maroto and David Pettinicchio, "Barriers to Economic Security: Disability, Employment, and Asset Disparities in Canada," *SSRN* (2020). papers.ssrn.com/sol3/papers.cfm?abstract_id=3532036.
8. Jonathan Pyzer, "Can You Get Charged for Reading Someone's E-Mail?" Toronto Defence Lawyers, August 7, 2021. torontodefencelawyers.com/can-get-charged-reading-someones-e-mail/.
9. Grant Cameron, "Industry Perspectives Op-Ed: COVID-19 Impact on Material Prices Creating Storm Clouds for Construction," *Construct Connect,* May 31, 2021. canada.constructconnect.com/dcn/news/resource/2021/05/industry-perspectives-op-ed-covid-19-impact-on-material-prices-creating-storm-clouds-for-construction.
10. Rachelle Elsiufi, "Homeowners Facing Major Backlog to Repair Damage from May 21 Storm." CBC News Online, June 4, 2022. cbc.ca/news/canada/ottawa/backlogs-to-repair-homes-after-storm-derecho-ottawa-1.6475400.
11. Aya Al-Hakim, "Nova Scotia Disability, Accessible Housing Advocate Passes Away at Age 47," *Global News,* May 24, 2019. globalnews.ca/news/5289049/nova-scotia-disability-advocate-passes-away; Robert Devet, "Joanne Larade, Disability Rights Advocate, Passes Away,"

Nova Scotia Advocate, May 20, 2019. nsadvocate.org/2019/05/20/
joanne-larade-disability-rights-advocate-passes-away/.

12. Victoria Levack, "Holiday Rules in Long-Term Care: An Open Letter
from Victoria Levack," *Disability Rights Coalition of Nova Scotia*,
December 24, 2021. disabilityrightscoalitionns.ca/2021/12/24/
holiday-rules-in-long-term-care-an-open-letter-from-victoria-levack/.

13. Vicky Levack and Megan Linton, "Fighting for the Right to Fuck,"
Briarpatch Magazine, September 7 2022. https://briarpatchmagazine.com/
articles/view/fighting-for-the-right-to-fuck.

14. Molly M. Perkin, Mary M. Ball, Frank J. Whittington et al. "Relational
Autonomy in Assisted Living: A Focus on Diverse Care Settings for
Older Adults," *Journal of Aging Studies,* 26, 1 (2012). doi.org/10.1016/j.
jaging.2012.01.001.

15. Adam Cotter and Laura Savage, *Gender-Based Violence and Unwanted
Sexual Behaviour in Canada, 2018: Initial Findings from the Survey of
Safety in Public and Private Spaces,* Statistics Canada, December 5, 2019.
www150.statcan.gc.ca/n1/en/pub/85-002-x/2019001/article/00017-eng.
pdf?st=C0qePEld.

16. Government of Nova Scotia, "Sexual Violence: A Public Health Primer,"
n.d. https://novascotia.ca/coms/svs/docs/primer.pdf.

17. National Center for Victims of Crime, "Crimes against People with
Disabilities," n.d. ncjrs.gov/ovc_archives/ncvrw/2017/images/en_artwork/
Fact_Sheets/2017NCVRW_PeopleWithDisabilities_508.pdf.

18. Kira S. Jones, "Attending to Our Needs: An Overview
of the Sexuality and Access Project," National Women's
Health Network, September 1, 2012. nwhn.org/
attending-to-our-needs-an-overview-of-the-sexuality-and-access-project/.

19. Steven J. Welch and Gerrit W. Clements, "Development of a
Policy on Sexuality for Hospitalized Chronic Psychiatric Patients,"
Canadian Journal of Psychiatry, 41, 5 (1996). https://doi.
org/10.1177/070674379604100503.

20. *New York Times,* "Sex and the Seniors: Survey Shows Many Elderly People
Remain Frisky," August 22, 2007. nytimes.com/2007/08/22/health/22iht-
22sex.7216942.html.

21. Mary-Catherine McIntosh, "'I Have Sex. Get Over It': Disability Activists
Call for Sex Education," *CBC News* (radio segment), October 30, 2017.
cbc.ca/radio/thecurrent/the-current-for-october-30-2017-1.4375925/i-
have-sex-get-over-it-disability-activists-call-for-sex-education-1.4375946.

22. Kirby Dick, *Private Practices: The Story of a Sex Surrogate,* Zeitgeist Films
(film), 1985. zeitgeistfilms.com/film/privatepractices; Ben Lewin, *The
Sessions,* Rhino Films (film), November 16, 2012.

23. Statistics Canada, *Census Profile, 2021 Census of Population, Profile Table,*
2021. https://www12.statcan.gc.ca/census-recensement/2021/dp-pd/prof/
details/page.cfm?Lang=E&SearchText=Nova%20Scotia&DGUIDlist=202

1A000212&GENDERlist=1,2,3&STATISTIClist=1&HEADERlist=0.

24. Janice Keefe, Cheryl, A. Smith and Greg Archibald, "Minister's Expert Advisory Panel on Long Term Care, Recommendations," Government of Nova Scotia, 2018. novascotia.ca/dhw/publications/Minister-Expert-Advisory-Panel-on-Long-Term-Care.pdf.

25. Carole A. Estabrooks, Sharon E. Straus, Colleen M. Flood et al. "Restoring Trust: COVID-19 and the Future of Long-Term Care in Canada." *FACETS*, August 27, 2020. facetsjournal.com/doi/10.1139/facets-2020-0056.

26. Kelly Fritsch and Fady Shanouda, "Warehousing Disabled People in Long-Term Care Homes Needs to Stop. Instead, Nationalize Home Care," *The Conversation*, January 12, 2022. theconversation.com/warehousing-disabled-people-in-long-term-care-homes-needs-to-stop-instead-nationalize-home-care-173412.

27. Locked Out of Life, "Tyson's Story," September 6, 2018. https://www.lockedoutoflife.com/stories/tysons-story/.

28. *CityNews*, "Staffing Shortages Cause Admissions Halt at 25 Nova Scotia Nursing Homes," January 11, 2022. https://halifax.citynews.ca/nova-scotia-news/staffing-shortages-cause-admissions-halt-at-25-nova-scotia-nursing-homes-4944131.

29. Government of Nova Scotia, "Continuing Care," n.d. novascotia.ca/dhw/ccs/policies-standards.asp.

30. Premier's Office, "Better Wages for Continuing Care Assistants," Government of Nova Scotia, February 9, 2022. novascotia.ca/news/release/?id=20220209006.

31. Interview by Lillian Cunningham, "Nurses, Fathers, Teachers, Mothers. Why Do We Devalue Someone the Minute They Care for Others?" *Washington Post*, October 21, 2021. washingtonpost.com/news/on-leadership/wp/2015/10/21/nurses-fathers-teachers-mothers-why-do-we-devalue-someone-the-minute-they-care-for-others/.

32. Jennifer Henderson, "Nursing Home Workers Are Moving between Multiple Facilities. That's a Big Problem," *Halifax Examiner*, April 17, 2020. https://www.halifaxexaminer.ca/province-house/nursing-home-workers-are-moving-between-multiple-facilities-thats-a-big-problem/.

Chapter 4

IT'S HAPPENING

In the 2022–23 Nova Scotia provincial budget, there is a provision that in the next calendar year 25 young adults who are currently in long-term care facilities, otherwise known as nursing homes, will be given the option of living in community. I talked to Vicky, who characteristically said we may have won the battle, but we haven't won the war. She said she will not rest until all younger adults are out of nursing homes and all institutions are closed. I don't know if I have the stamina for that. For now, I will celebrate the victory no matter how incomplete it may be. I tell myself at least we are on the premier's radar, and we have shaken up a system that is 50 years behind what is happening on the other coast.

I received an email from Maria Medioli, the executive director of the Disability Support Program with the NS Department of Community Services, inviting me to the budget lock-up at the end of March. She said I was going to receive an official invitation, but she wanted to give me a heads up. At the time I was barely keeping my head above water; my partner Tom, who since the onset of COVID-19 had been my primary caregiver, had fallen out of bed and fractured a vertebra in his spine. He had just returned to sleeping with me after spending a week in the spare bedroom. I was worried about when he had to come off the painkillers because the doctor had prescribed oxycodone and, according to my friend who is a musician and knows more about substances than he probably should, "oxy is a bitch to come off of." I was interested in why

Maria thought the lock-up would be of interest to me. I had gone to budget lock-ups when I was working for Nova Scotia League for Equal Opportunities and again when I was working for the Ecology Action Centre.

On March 30, 2022, I sent Maria Medioli the following email:

> I am sorry I did not make it to lock-up yesterday. My partner (Tom) who has been doing all of my homecare fractured a vertebra three weeks ago. He is walking fine after using a walker for a week. He is using the microwave and oven now, while for the first two weeks he ate only canned food. But he is not at the point where he can get me dressed and put me in my wheelchair. I am sorry I couldn't make the lock-up. I was reading the summary, and I was wondering if you think I have mental health concerns. There was a lot of money for that.

I received the following email back:

> Great to hear from you Jen. I admit I was a touch worried when I didn't see you there. Buried in all the new health and mental health dollars is an additional $27.0 million to move an additional 200 young people out of long-term care into community using the shared services model over the next four years (25 placements this year). I am so happy! You should be so proud, if it wasn't for you this would not be happening. I can't wait to get moving on this!

The work that needed to be done to implement the Shared Attendant Program was monumental. The policy regarding the care of people with "complex care needs" in the Nova Scotia government had remained unchanged for the past 50 years. This new pilot of the Shared Attendant Care program modified all that.

Nova Scotia was no longer going to be the backward neighbour. It was going to be cutting edge. Nova Scotia will always be the last province to close its institutions, but it need not be a disappointment in all respects.

125

ACKNOWLEDGEMENTS

I want to thank all of the assistants who wrote with me. I know it was tedious, but I couldn't have done it without you: Calisse, Farzan, Rae, Emily, Isaac, Sonya and Abby. I also want to thank Abby for introducing me to partner assisted scanning; it is helpful to hire students. If you had already written your licensing exam, I would have to pay for your knowledge. I want to thank Carrie and Kathleen for reviewing my chaplets. I want to thank Vicky for adding her voice through endless interviews. I want to thank Leah for answering my questions. I would like to thank the Dave Greber Freelance Writers Awards. The close of the competition was at the same time as my writing deadline so I do not know if my submission was chosen. But winning is immaterial, the fact that the award exists is motivation enough. It reminds writers that what they do is important. I would like to thank Global Television Network for the article on Joanne Larade. I want to thank Fernwood and all its staff for believing in the project. This has been quite the journey. Thank you for travelling with me.